Avoiding Errors in
General Practice

Avoiding Errors in
General Practice

Kevin Barraclough

MA, FRCP, FRCGP, LLB
General Practitioner
Painswick Surgery, Painswick
Gloucestershire, UK

Jenny du Toit

FRCP, FRCGP
General Practitioner
Painswick Surgery, Painswick
Gloucestershire, UK

Jeremy Budd

MB, Bchir, FRCGP
General Practitioner
East Quay Medical Centre
Bridgwater, Somerset, UK

Joseph E. Raine

MD, FRCPCH, DCH
Consultant Paediatrician
Whittington Hospital
London, UK

Kate Williams

MA (Oxon)
Partner
Radcliffes LeBrasseur Solicitors
Leeds, UK

Jonathan Bonser

BA (Oxon)
Consultant in the Healthcare Department of
Fishburns LLP, Solicitors
London, UK
Former Head of the Claims and Legal Services
Department of the Leeds office of the Medical Protection Society

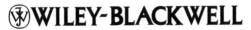

WILEY-BLACKWELL

A John Wiley & Sons, Ltd., Publication

Wiley-Blackwell is an imprint of John Wiley & Sons, formed by the merger of Wiley's global Scientific, Technical and Medical business with Blackwell Publishing.

Registered office: John Wiley & Sons, Ltd, The Atrium, Southern Gate, Chichester, West Sussex, PO19 8SQ, UK

Editorial offices: 9600 Garsington Road, Oxford, OX4 2DQ, UK

The Atrium, Southern Gate, Chichester, West Sussex, PO19 8SQ, UK

111 River Street, Hoboken, NJ 07030-5774, USA

For details of our global editorial offices, for customer services and for information about how to apply for permission to reuse the copyright material in this book please see our website at www.wiley.com/wiley-blackwell.

Library of Congress Cataloging-in-Publication Data

Avoiding errors in general practice / Kevin Barraclough ... [et al.].
      p. ; cm.
   Includes bibliographical references and index.
   ISBN 978-0-470-67357-7 (pbk. : alk. paper)
   I. Barraclough, Kevin.
   [DNLM: 1. Medical Errors–legislation & jurisprudence–Case Reports.   2. Medical Errors–prevention & control–Case Reports.   3. General Practice–organization & administration–Case Reports.   4. Primary Health Care–organization & administration–Case Reports. WB 100]

610.28′9–dc23   2012031977

A catalogue record for this book is available from the British Library.

Wiley also publishes its books in a variety of electronic formats. Some content that appears in print may not be available in electronic books.

Cover Design: Sarah Dickinson

Set in 10.5/13 pt Minion by Aptara® Inc., New Delhi, India

1   2013

Contents

Part 2 Clinical cases

Part 3 Investigating and dealing with errors

Contributors

Joanne Haswell
Barrister; Director, InPractice Training
London
Part 1, Section 3

Nicola Hayward
Practice Manager; Hoyland House Surgery,
Painswick
Part 1, Section 3

Alistair Hewitt
Partner, Radcliffes LeBrasseur
Leeds
Section 3: Coroner's court, Criminal matters

Kate Hill
Solicitor, Radcliffes LeBrasseur
Managing Director, InPractice Training,
London
Part 1, Section 3

Preface

Like most general practitioners, I am anxious about being sued. It is clearly necessary to have such a process in society to right clinical 'wrongs', but as a doctor it is difficult to be very enthusiastic about it.

However, negligence cases – whether justified or not – do provide an extraordinarily rich source of material from which to improve one's clinical practice. I have learnt a great deal over the last decade of examining such cases, and it has certainly changed my practice.

I have learnt to be very wary about the spectrum of presentations of those conditions that come up recurrently in medico-legal practice – appendicitis, ischaemic feet, subarachnoid haemorrhages, pulmonary emboli etc. The 40 case studies in Part 2 cover over 95% of all conditions that end in litigation against general practitioners.

I suspect that an awareness that I could be sued does also encourage me to second guess my clinical reasoning – 'could I be wrong here?' That process is, I think, an essential part of being a good clinician. Part 1 examines in more detail the techniques which help a clinician to avoid errors.

Being a good general practitioner is, as we all know, difficult. There is a fine line between being over cautious (and medicalizing everyone) – and being under cautious (and missing serious illness). I hope this book provides some help in walking that tightrope. Part 3 provides some guidance if you fall off the tightrope!

Kevin Barraclough
Painswick, UK

Abbreviations

A&E	Accident & Emergency	DKA	Diabetic ketoacidosis
ABPI	Ankle Brachial Pressure Index	DOH	Department of Health
ACE	Angiotensin converting enzyme	DRE	Digital rectal examination
ACS	Acute coronary syndrome	DVT	Deep vein thrombosis
ALT	Alanine transaminase	ECG	Electrocardiogram
AMUSE	Amsterdam Maastricht Utrecht study on safety and cost-effectiveness of a diagnostic decision rule for suspected deep venous thrombosis in general practice.	ED	Emergency Department
		ELISA	Enzyme-linked immunosorbent assay
		ESR	Erythrocyte sedimentation rate
		FBC	Full blood count
		FOBs	Faecal occult bloods
AST	Aspartate transaminase	GCA	Giant cell arteritis
βhCG	Beta human chorionic gonadatrophin	GMC	General Medical Council
		GORD	Gastro oesophageal reflux disease
BJGP	British Journal of General Practice	GP	General practitioner
BMI	Body mass index	GPRD	General Practice Research Database
BMJ	British Medical Journal		
BNF	British National Formulary	GTN	Glyceryl trinitrate
BP	Blood pressure	Hb	Haemoglobin
BPPV	Benign paroxysmal positional vertigo	HCG/L	Human chorionic gonadatrophin per litre
BSG	British Society of Gastroenterology	HIV	Human Immunodeficiency Virus
BTA	British Thyroid Association	HPA	Heath Protection Agency
BTS	British Thoracic Society	HSC	Health Service Commissioner
BUPA	British United Provident Association	IMB	Intermenrtrual bleeding
		ICU	Intensive care unit
CAP	Community Acquired Pneumonia	IOP	Interim Orders Panel
		IT	Intrathecal
CBE	Clinical breast examination	ITU	Intensive therapy unit
CDH	Congenital Dislocation of the Hip	IV	Intravenous
		JAMA	Journal of the American Medical Association
CES	Cauda equina syndrome		
CKD	Chroinc kidney disease	LFT	Liver function test
COCP	Combined oral contraceptive	LR−	negative likelihood ratio
CPR	Clinical Prediction Rules	LR +	positive likelihood ratio
CPS	Crown Prosecution Service	MCV	Mean corpuscular volume
CRC	Colorectal cancer	MDDUS	Medical and Dental Defence Union of Scotland
CRP	C-reactive protein		
CRT	Capillary return time	MDOs	Medical Defence Organizations
CT	Computerised tomography	MDU	Medical Defence Union
DDH	Developmental Displasia of the Hip	MPS	Medical Protection Society
		MRI	Magnetic resonance imaging
DGH	District general hospital	MSU	Mid stream urine

NAD	Nothing abnormal detected	PR	Per rectum
NCAS	National Clinical Assessment Service	PSA	Prostate specific antigen
		PTSD	post-traumatic distress
NEMC-PCR	New England Medical Centre Posterior Circulation Registry	RCP	Royal College of Physicians
		SAH	Subarachnoid haemorrhage
NHS	National Health Service	SEA	Significant Event Analysis
NHSLA	NHS Litigation Authority	SHO	Senior House Officer
NICE	National Institute for Clinical Excellence	SnOUT	when a **sen**sitive test is **n**egative, it rules the diagnosis **out**
NNT	Numbers needed to treat	SOAP	Subject, Object, Assessment, Plan
NSAIDs	Non-steroidal anti inflammatory drugs	Sp	Specificity
O/E	On examination	SpIN	when a **sp**ecific test is **p**ositive, it rules the diagnosis **in**
OOH	Out of Hours	SUFE	slipped upper femoral epiphysis
OSCE	Objective Structure Clinical Examination	TFT	Thyroid function test
		TIA	Transient ischaemic attack
PCB	Post-coital bleeding	TPO	Thyroid peroxidise
PCRS	Primary Care Respiratory Society	TSH	Thyroid stimulating hormone
PCTs	Primary Care Trusts	U&E	Urea & electrolytes
PE	Pulmonary embolism	UTI	Urinary tract infection
PEFR	Peak expiratory flow rate		
PIOPED	Prospective Investigation of Pulmonary Embolism Diagnosis study		

Introduction

In 2000, a committee established by the Department of Health, chaired by the then Chief Medical Officer, Professor Liam Donaldson, published its report *An Organisation with a Memory*. The report recognized that the vast majority of NHS care was of a very high clinical standard and that serious failures were uncommon, given the volume of care provided. However, when failures do occur their consequences can be devastating for the individual patients and their families. The healthcare workers feel guilt and distress. Like a ripple effect, the mistakes also undermine the public's confidence in the health service. Last, but not least, these adverse events have a huge cumulative financial effect. Updating the figures provided in the report, in 2010/11, the NHS Litigation Authority (the NHSLA is the body that handles negligence claims against NHS Trusts in England) paid out nearly £863 000 000 for medical negligence claims (these figures take no account of the costs incurred by the Medical Defence Organisations for General Practice and private health care). The report commented ruefully that often these failures have a familiar ring to them; many could be avoided 'if only the lessons of experience were properly learned'.

The Committee writing the report also noted that there is a vast reservoir of clinical data from negligence claims that remains untapped. They were gently critical of the Health Service as being par excellence a passive learning organization; like a school teacher writing an end of term report, they classified the NHS a poor learner – could do better. On a more positive note, the report stated that 'There is significant potential to extract valuable learning by focusing, specialty by specialty, on the main areas of practice that have resulted in litigation.' It acknowledged that learning from adverse clinical events is a key component of clinical governance and is an important component in delivering the government's quality agenda for the NHS.

The NHSLA has reported that its present (as of 2011) estimate for all potential liabilities, existing and expected claims, is £16.8 billion. At the time *An Organisation with a Memory* was written, this figure stood at £2.4 billion. (These sums are actuarially calculated figures that are based on both known and as yet unknown claims, some of which may not surface for many years to come. They should not be confused with the figure of £863 000 000 mentioned above, which was the sum actually paid out in one year.) The NHSLA also reported that the number of negligence claims rose from 6652 in 2009/10 to 8655 in 2010/11. While the increases in these figures may be due to the increased readiness of patients to pursue negligence claims and the very significant costs of claims inflation, rather than any marked decline in the standard of care provided by the NHS, the statistics clearly show that there is still room for improvement in the care provided to patients. It is this gap in the standard of care that we, the authors, wish to address through this book, and the series of which it is a part.

An Organisation with a Memory as a report tried to take a fresh look at the nature of mistakes within the NHS. It looked at fields of activity outside health care, such as the airline industry. The committee commented that there were two ways of viewing human error: the person-centred approach and the systems approach. The person-centred approach focuses on the individual, his inattention, forgetfulness and carelessness. Its correctives are aimed at individuals and propagate a blame culture. The systems approach, on the other hand, takes a holistic view of the reasons for failure. It recognizes that many of the problems facing large organizations are complex and result from the interplay of many factors: errors often arise from the cumulative effect of a number of small mistakes; they cannot always be pinned on one blameworthy individual. This approach starts from the position that humans do make mistakes and that errors are inevitable, but tries to change the environment in which people work, so that fewer mistakes will be made.

The systems approach does not, however, absolve individuals of their responsibilities. Rather, it suggests that we should not automatically assume that we should look for an individual to blame for an adverse outcome. The authors of *An Organisation with a Memory* acknowledged that clinical practice did differ from many hi-tech industries. The airline industry, for example, can place a number of hi-tech safeguards between danger and harm. This is often not possible in many fields of clinical practice, where the human elements are often the last and the most important defences. 'In surgery,' they wrote, 'very little lies between the scalpel and some untargeted nerve or blood vessel other than the skill and training of the surgeon.' We believe that this difference is key to understanding the nature of error in healthcare and why we have placed such great emphasis on case studies that show how doctors make mistakes in treating their patients.

The committee felt that the NHS had for too long taken a person-centred approach to the errors made by its employees and that this had stifled improvement. They called for a change in the culture of the NHS and a move away from what they saw as its blame culture. More than a decade has passed since the writing of the report and there has been little change in attitudes. A sea change is required. We want to see an NHS that promotes a safety culture, rather than a blame culture, a culture where there are multiple safeguards built into the system.

However, the legal system in which the medical services operate does not foster such an approach. Although coroners can now comment on the strengths and weaknesses of systems in the form of narrative verdicts, in general, the medical complaints and litigation process still tends to focus on the actions of individuals rather than the failings of the system. Perhaps the most glaring example of this person-centred approach can be seen in the way the General Medical Council treats medical practitioners, when they receive a complaint. In that forum, doctors are expected to meet personal professional standards and will be held to account if they fall short of them in any way. Yet they may find themselves working in an environment that at times seems to conflict with those professional standards.

In Reason (2000) Professor James Reason (originator of the well known 'Swiss Cheese' explanation of how errors sometimes lead to damage) stated:

> The longstanding and widespread tradition of the person approach focuses on the unsafe acts – errors and procedural violations – of people at the sharp end: nurses, physicians, surgeons, anaesthetists, pharmacists, and the like. It views these unsafe acts as arising primarily from aberrant mental processes such as forgetfulness, inattention, poor motivation, carelessness, negligence, and recklessness. Naturally enough, the associated countermeasures are directed mainly at reducing unwanted variability in human behaviour. These methods include poster campaigns that appeal to people's sense of fear, writing another procedure (or adding to existing ones), disciplinary measures, threat of litigation, retraining, naming, blaming, and shaming. Followers of this approach tend to treat errors as moral issues, assuming that bad things happen to bad people – what psychologists have called the just world hypothesis.
>
> The basic premise in the system approach is that humans are fallible and errors are to be expected, even in the best organisations. Errors are seen as consequences rather than causes, having their origins not so much in the perversity of human nature as in 'upstream' systemic factors. These include recurrent error traps in the workplace and the organisational processes that give rise to them. Countermeasures are based on the assumption that though we cannot change the human condition, we can change the conditions under which humans work. A central idea is that of system defences. All hazardous technologies possess barriers and safeguards. When an adverse event occurs, the important issue is not who blundered, but how and why the defences failed. (Reproduced from J. Reason (2000) Human error: models and management, *BMJ* 320:768, with permission from BMJ Publishing Group Ltd.)

As authors, we believe that the Committee of *An Organisation with a Memory* were right when they wrote that many useful lessons can be learnt from the bitter experience of errors and litigation and that this can best be done by looking specialty by specialty at those areas of practice where errors are most frequently made. Thus, we have produced a book looking at errors in general practice. It will fit into a series of such books, each concentrating on a separate specialty.

If doctors are to learn lessons from their errors and litigation, then they must have some understanding of the underlying processes. Thus, in Part 1, Section 1 we discuss the key legal concepts and how they interact with medical practice. We will examine the document *An Organisation with a Memory*, published in 2000. This was the report of an expert group on learning from adverse events in the NHS that was chaired by the Chief Medical Officer. One hospital negligence case was examined in some detail to identify how system failures contribute to personal error. We will look at that case briefly.

Most litigation cases in general practice concern failure to diagnose or delay in diagnosis or referral. In Part 1, Section 2, we will examine aspects that contribute to this. We will look at evidence about how general practitioners reach diagnoses, and evidence about where cognitive errors arise. We will suggest a simple six-step strategy for minimizing those risks.

In Part 1, Section 3, we will briefly examine how Bayesian reasoning can illuminate the process of clinical reasoning and where the errors are likely to occur. We will examine 'SnOUTs' and 'SpINs' and likelihood ratios (these will be explained later!).

In Part 1, Section 4, we will examine a potpourri of issues that lead to errors: problems with the history and examination, telephone consultations, communication problems, knowledge failures, the unexpectedly abnormal result, note-keeping, drug or prescribing errors and the issue of consent. We will flag up 'frequent fliers' in negligence cases and how to avoid them. Lastly, we will deal with the crucial aspect of 'safety netting'.

The heart of the book is in fact in Part 2. Here, we set out a number of case studies on common mistakes in general practice. Each case is drawn from real scenarios, anonymized to protect patient confidentiality and is supplemented with legal comment. Most cases concern failures to diagnose an illness, the commonest source of error in medical treatment and the commonest cause of litigation against general practitioners.

Finally, Part 3 provides a practical guide to the various forms of complaint that a general practitioner may encounter, how they may affect her and what she can do to protect her interests (gender pronouns will be used indiscriminately!).

Our aim is to provide a book that will go some way to meet the challenges laid down at the turn of the millennium in *An Organisation with a Memory*. We hope that it will reduce the number of clinical errors and improve the standard of care provided by individual general practitioners and practices throughout the country.

References and further reading

Department of Health (2000) An Organisation with a Memory, the report of an expert group on learning from adverse events in the NHS, chaired by the Chief Medical Officer (2000). http://www.dh.gov.uk/en/Publication sandstatistics/Publications/PublicationsPolicyAndGuidance/DH_4065083

Reason J (2000) In human error: models and management. *BMJ* **320**: 768–70.

Section 1: The legal structure of negligence

A few words about error

If our aim is to reduce the number of clinical errors, then we must explain what we mean by 'error'. The Oxford English Dictionary defines 'an error' as a mistake. This is self-evident and does not really help us, the authors, to define our goal.

We could define our aim by looking at the end-result of errors and say that we want to prevent poor patient outcomes. That must be our primary concern, but our aim is broader; many mistakes can be rectified before any serious harm is done.

We could look at the seriousness of the error, how 'bad' the mistake actually was. Some errors could be so crass and the consequences so serious that they can be labelled 'criminal' by one and all and in fact some cases are investigated by the police and come before the criminal courts, as we shall see later. Other errors are the sort that only become obvious with the benefit of hindsight and could be made by anyone, even the best of doctors. In short, we want to look at all errors across the spectrum. What we hope to achieve is to raise the standard of care provided to patients, so that mistakes of all kinds are reduced.

But as soon as we mention error, the word negligence also springs to mind. The law has defined negligence in specific terms and not all errors will be considered negligent. But since the law looms large in any discussion of clinical error, we will now provide a brief explanation of what negligence in a legal context actually means and on how the compensation that we mentioned in our Introduction is calculated, when negligence occurs.

Medical negligence

If a doctor makes a mistake in the treatment of a patient, then he or in the case of a child, his family, may decide to pursue the doctor for compensation. Generally speaking, in order to win compensation, the family will have to prove that the doctor (or the collectively the practice, or Trust) were negligent.

Negligence

Before looking in detail at what is relevant to this book, medical negligence, we need to know the basics that lie behind what is called the tort of negligence

Avoiding Errors in General Practice, First Edition. Kevin Barraclough, Jenny du Toit, Jeremy Budd, Joseph E. Raine, Kate Williams and Jonathan Bonser.
© 2013 John Wiley & Sons, Ltd. Published 2013 by John Wiley & Sons, Ltd.

(tort is simply the old French word for wrong; in modern legal terms, it forms a branch of legal study).

In principle, a person is liable in negligence if he breaches a duty owed to another in such a way as to cause damage to that person. What does this mean? In practical terms, in order to decide whether an act is negligent, a lawyer will break this formula down, looking at each of its constituent parts, phrase by phrase, word by word. For example, he will ask himself whether a duty of care exists between the injured person and the alleged defendant.

It may not always be clear whether a duty exists in a given set of circumstances, but as far as medical treatment is concerned, it is assumed that a doctor owes such a duty to his patient. The key questions in any medical negligence case are whether that duty to take care has been breached and then if it has, whether any damage has been caused as a result of that breach.

Has there been a breach of duty?

When the treatment of a patient comes under scrutiny in a potential negligence claim, the first question that will be asked is: was that treatment in accordance with the standards of a body of reasonable or responsible general practitioners? If it was, then the general practitioner will not have breached their duty of care; but if the treatment does not accord with the standards of a reasonable body of general practitioners, then they will have breached that duty.

This test was first formulated by the House of Lords in the case of *Bolam v Friern Hospital Management Committee* in 1957. Hence the *Bolam* test.

Over the years, a body of cases has built up that indicates how this *Bolam* test should be applied. How, for instance, should we look on a case, where in a given set of circumstances, one set of general practitioners may treat a patient in a certain fashion, while others would adopt a different approach? Answer: it is enshrined in case law that so long as both bodies of general practitioners are reasonable/responsible, then it would not matter which of the two approaches the doctor adopted. In other words, it is possible to have more than one correct approach to treatment.

But this begs the question: who determines whether you have breached your duty of care?

If a general practitioner has received a letter of claim from the solicitors representing the family concerning the treatment of a patient, this should indicate that the family have investigated the case and gone to medical experts who have written reports critical of the care provided. At first blush, there is a case for the doctor to answer.

In response, the defence organization of the general practitioner, or the lawyers for the Trust, will instruct experts to look at the allegations made against it. The experts will be asked to consider both breach of duty and causation. So in the first instance, the answer to the question is that the opinions of the experts, as interpreted by the lawyers, will determine the progress of the case. If both experts, the expert for the family and the expert for the defendant believe that the care was substandard (it did not accord with the standards of a reasonable body of general practitioners), then it is likely that the defence organization will concede that the treating doctor has breached their duty of care. But what happens, if the expert for the defendant general practitioner concludes that the treating clinicians have not breached their duty of care?

At this point one may say that the difference in the two opinions, that of the family's expert and that of the defendant's expert, simply reflects two different approaches. Have we not just said that a doctor will not breach his duty of care, so long as he acts in accordance with a reasonable body of opinion? Has not the general practitioner's expert supported the clinicians' care? Is this not enough?

The short answer is that it may be, but not necessarily. The *Bolam* test has been qualified or rather refined by the case of *Bolitho v City and Hackney Health Authority*. The judges in this 1993 case stated that although one group of so called reasonable practitioners may adopt a certain approach to treatment, if that approach does not stand up to logical analysis, then a doctor cannot expect his treatment of the patient to be endorsed, if he adopted that apparently 'reasonable', but illogical approach to treatment. This is just one way in which the competing views of experts may be resolved. But it may come down to something less tangible: merely that one expert is more believable than another.

At the end of the day, if the case cannot be determined by other means, it will come before a judge, who will hear all the evidence, listen to the experts and decide which of them he prefers. It is, of course, he who will be the final arbiter. But before then, depending upon where in the United Kingdom the case is brought (the procedural rules differ from jurisdiction to jurisdiction), evidence will have been disclosed, meetings will be held and views will crystallize. The experts for the opposing sides will have met and their opinions may shift one way or the other. The reality is that few cases will go before a judge. They will either be settled out of court or the patient or family will decide to drop the case.

Causation

But let us assume that the patient proves that the general practitioner has breached their duty of care to him or her. This does not automatically mean that they will be awarded any money. In order to obtain compensation, they must clear the causation hurdle. They must demonstrate that the breach of duty caused some injury or damage to them, that it changed the outcome for the worse.

In some cases, causation is uncomplicated and straightforward. In others, it can be fiendishly complex. In the context of this book, we shall not delve too deeply into its intricacies, but hope to give you some idea of its basic concepts.

As an example of straightforward causation, take the case of a general practitioner who misdiagnoses acute angle closure glaucoma as migraine and the patient loses the use of one eye. It will be relatively easy to prove causation because if the condition was suspected and diagnosed while the patient had a painful eye but good sight, swift treatment would have saved the sight.

Causation will be far less easy to prove in a case of delayed diagnosis of colorectal cancer. At diagnosis the patient had inoperable disease with distant metastases. Would the metastases still have been there if the general practitioner had referred the patient 9 months earlier? The patient died of his disease, but would he have lived but for the delay?

Damages

The purpose of a claim in negligence is to provide the patient or family with compensation for any harm done to him through substandard care. Once it is established that the doctor has breached his duty of care to the patient and that that breach has caused injury, the court will move on to determine how much the claimant should be awarded in damages.

Clearly, it is impossible to adequately compensate someone in monetary terms for the physical disabilities they may suffer as a result of negligence, but the idea behind compensation is to put the patient or family in the same position as they would have been, if the error had not been made.

The patient will be given a sum of money which is designed to compensate him for his pain and suffering. He will also receive a sum to compensate him for any monetary expense arising from the negligence which he has incurred in the past: for example, the costs of physiotherapy.

Finally, he will be compensated for the future losses that he will incur as a result of the negligence. The sorts of loss will depend on the severity of the injury. In the most severe cases of brain damage, the compensation for future loss could include sums for loss of earnings, the cost of buying and adapting a suitable home, the costs of nursing care, physiotherapy, occupational therapy, speech therapy and computer technology to aid in communication. Over the lifetime of a brain-damaged child, for example, the loss that he will suffer as a result of negligence could easily be several million pounds, depending on his life expectancy.

The claimant may receive the damages as a one-off lump sum payment. Alternatively, he may receive periodical payments spread over his lifetime.

If, however, the patient dies as a result of negligence, then the damages will be very limited. His estate will be awarded a sum for his pain and suffering and his funeral expenses. The family will also receive a statutory sum for bereavement damages that is currently set at £11 800.

The limitation period

An adult injured through medical negligence has three years to start his claim formally in the courts. (This three year period runs essentially from the time when the negligence occurred, but is more accurately defined by when the person harmed knew of the negligence.) Although the court can extend this limitation period in certain circumstances, if he fails to start court proceedings within these three years, he can no longer pursue his claim.

The rules concerning children are different. Children are not considered to have legal capacity until they are 18. Before then, a child's case will be brought on his behalf by his parents, standing in the child's legal shoes. The 'limitation clock' does not start to tick until the 18th birthday. Therefore, a child who has suffered injury has until he is 21 to bring a claim.

However, if a person lacks mental capacity beyond the age of 18, the limitation clock may never start to run. He can then bring a case at any point in his life. 'Mental capacity' in this context means the ability to run one's own financial affairs; it is different from the test for capacity in consent cases (see below).

The most expensive cases, the ones that cost millions of pounds, are often those that concern brain-damaged infants from the most severe cases to those suffering some form of developmental delay (e.g. through an alleged delay in diagnosing and treating meningitis). It is not unusual for these cases to be litigated 20, 30 or more years after the date of the alleged negligence. This may seem strange. There are several reasons why this may be so. But the family often only discover the true difficulties of looking after a brain-damaged child when the child grows older and his lack of mobility becomes a problem and it may be only then that their thoughts turn to suing the clinical team that treated their child. Or it may be that the family's lawyer will advise them to delay the claim until the impact of the injury on the child and family can be fully assessed.

When a patient dies, whether a child or an adult, his personal representatives will have three years to start proceedings. This three years runs from the date of death or when it was known that there had been a mistake, if this is later.

Jurisdictions

The United Kingdom is divided into a number of different legal jurisdictions. In certain areas of law, England and Wales, Scotland and Northern Ireland have their own, different set of rules, as do also the Channel Islands and the Isle of Man. However, what we have said above about medical negligence applies to all jurisdictions. (The Scottish word for tort is delict, but the principles are the same.) However, these jurisdictions do have their own rules for procedure, that affect how a case is litigated.

The defence of the NHS trusts in medical negligence cases is also organized in different ways. Thus the NHSLA is responsible for cases in England, whereas

Welsh Health Legal services is responsible in Wales. In essence, however, defence of such cases is financed out of central funds, no matter where in the United Kingdom NHS hospital cases are litigated. General practitioners are generally represented by one or other of the Medical Defence Organisations (MDOs): either the MDU, MPS or the MDDUS.

Learning from system failures – the vincristine example

The way that the courts look at negligence is to focus on the acts of individuals and to ascribe fault to particular doctors, if their treatment of the patient fell below the standard of the *Bolam* test. But as mentioned in our Introduction, there is another way of looking at errors and that is to consider system failures.

In order to illustrate the difference between system failures and individual fault, the authors of *An Organisation with a Memory* examined a case concerning the maladministration of the drug vincristine. The mistake cost the patient, a child, his life. A number of shortcomings occurred during the child's stay in the hospital. The events obviously occurred in hospital but the detailed analysis in the report shows well the generic mix of system and personal errors that lead to medical tragedies. We believe that it would be useful to set out what happened in the lead up to this child's death, pointing out at each stage, the failings that occurred. We will then provide a more detailed discussion of the general lessons that can be learnt from the case, and its applicability to medical mistakes in general.

The following is taken with minor amendment from *An Organisation with a Memory*. It is a classic example of how a number of small mistakes can add up to a massive error and end with a fatality. The comments in italics provide a brief analysis of the faults that occurred:

A child was being treated in a district general hospital (DGH). He was due to receive chemotherapy under a general anaesthetic at a specialist centre. He should have been fasted for 6 hours prior to the anaesthetic, but was allowed to eat and drink before leaving the DGH.
Fasting error. Poor communication between the DGH and the specialist centre.

When he arrived at the specialist centre, there were no beds available on the oncology ward, so he was admitted to a mixed-specialty 'outlier' ward.

Lack of organizational resources; there were no beds available for specialized treatment. The patient was placed in an environment where the staff had no specialist oncology expertise.

The patient's notes were lost and were not available to the ward staff on admission.
Loss of patient information.

The patient was due to receive intravenous vincristine, to be administered by a specialist oncology nurse on the ward, and intrathecal (spinal) methotrexate, to be administered in the operating theatre by an oncology Specialist Registrar. No oncology nurse specialist was available on the ward.

Communication failure between the oncology department and the outlier ward. Absence of policy and resources to deal with the demands placed on the system by outlier wards, including shortage of specialist staff.

Vincristine and methotrexate were transported together to the ward by a house-keeper instead of being kept separate at all times.

Drug delivery error due to noncompliance with hospital policy, which was that the drugs must be kept separate at all times. Communication error: the outlier ward was not aware of this policy.

The housekeeper who took the drugs to the ward informed staff that both drugs were to go to theatre with the patient.

Communication error. Incorrect information communicated. Poor delivery practice, allowing drugs to be delivered to outlier wards by inexperienced staff.

The patient was consented by a junior doctor. He was consented only for in-trathecal (IT) methotrexate and not for intravenous vincristine.

Poor consenting practice. Junior doctor allowed to take consent. Consenting error.

A junior doctor abbreviated the route of administration to IV and IT, instead of using the full term in capital letters.

Poor prescribing practice.

When the fasting error was discovered, the chemotherapy procedure was post-poned from the morning to the afternoon list. The doctor who had been due to administer the intrathecal drug had booked the afternoon off and assumed that another doctor in charge of the wards that day would take over. No formal face-to-face handover was carried out between the two doctors.

Communication failure. Poor handover of task responsibilities. Inappropriate task delegation.

The patient arrived in the anaesthetic room and the oncology Senior Registrar was called to administer the chemotherapy. However the doctor was unable to leave his ward and assured the anaesthetist that he should go ahead as this was a straight-forward procedure.

Inadequate protocols regulating the administration of high toxicity drugs. Goal conflict between ward and theatre duties. Poor practice expecting the doctor to be in two places at the same time.

The oncology Senior Registrar was not aware that both drugs had been delivered to theatre. The anaesthetist had the expertise to administer drugs intrathecally

but had never administered chemotherapy. He injected the methotrexate in-
travenously and the vincristine into the patient's spine. Intrathecal injection of
vincristine is almost invariably fatal, and the patient died 5 days later.
Situational awareness error. Inappropriate task delegation and lack of training.
Poor practice to allow chemotherapy drugs to be administered by someone with no
oncology experience. Drug administration error.

Although the authors of *An Organisation with a Memory* analyze this sorry
tale in the context of system failures, rather than individual fault, it is clear
that many of the failings represent a mixture of the two. Many of the actions
undertaken by an individual member of the hospital staff could be analyzed
in terms of the *Bolam* reasonableness test and be found wanting, i.e. the
individual would be found to be in breach of his duty of care to the child.
But that is not the point. The systems approach suggests that we should not
automatically assume that we should look for an individual to blame for an
adverse outcome. What we are asking is that when an error is made, the finger
should not necessarily be pointed at the doctor who made the final error. We
are asking that a more considered approach be taken that looks at matters in
the round, that digs a little deeper and tests the role of management and the
systems that operate in the hospital.

In a case such as this, a judge in the civil courts will most generally look at
the act that immediately *caused* the death, the intrathecal administration of
vincristine. It was the anaesthetist who did this and so a judge will focus his
attention on him. In terms of strict legal causation, most of the other failings
cannot be said to have caused the death. For example, the fact that the child's
notes went missing is clearly substandard and forms part of the background
circumstances that led to the fatal error. But the causal link between the loss
of the notes and the death is not strong.

As we approach in time the moment when the fatal dose was administered,
matters become less clear in terms of causation. The actions of the oncology
Senior Registrar – who, in having the afternoon off, failed to do a proper
handover – may not have directly caused the death. However, it is clear that
partly as a result of his omission, an inexperienced anaesthetist was put in a
situation in which he should not have found himself.

A poor handover is a systems error as well as an individual fault. It is clear
that the individual doctor had a lax attitude towards handover; he was dealing
with a child requiring specialist oncology treatment on an outlier ward. But it
is probably also representative of a systemic problem in the hospital. It could
be indicative of a lax attitude to this important element of patient care among
the hospital staff at large. Such statements are difficult to substantiate without
direct knowledge of how hospital was organized more than 10 years ago. But
what we do know is that the hospital failed in its treatment of this child.
The patient was placed on an outlier ward with no cover from a specialist
oncology nurse. There should have been a protocol in place to deal with
this situation.

Whether a civil court recognizes such errors or not, system failures do play their part in most cases of negligence; they produce the circumstances in which the final error is made.

Although the errors committed in this maladministration of vincristine are, of course, specific to the case, they also illustrate general issues and a number of themes emerge that warrant further discussion.

Failure to follow protocols or guidelines

A number of errors that occurred in the management of this child arose from either a failure to follow protocols or the absence of policy on key issues. Thus the housekeeper transported the vincristine and the methotrexate to the ward together; hospital policy was that the two drugs should have been kept separate at all times. When the patient was admitted to the outlier ward, there was no specialist oncology nurse to attend to his needs; there was no policy in place to deal with the demands of outlier wards, especially in relation to the availability of specialist staff.

The decade since the writing of *An Organisation with a Memory* has seen the introduction of numerous guidelines to try to improve the service offered by the hospitals and general practitioners to its patients. In hospital they will often be protocols. In general practice they will often be management or referral guidelines. These can only be for the good, setting in place good working practices and, therefore, improving patient care.

A general practitioner can take some comfort that by adhering to a guideline he may well be protected from criticism. In principle, a guideline issued by a respectable source can be regarded as a statement by a responsible body of medical opinion on what to do in a particular set of circumstances. But adherence may not always provide protection to a doctor. There may be some circumstance relevant to the individual patient that renders a particular guideline inappropriate. A guideline or protocol should not replace good judgement.

Whether a failure to follow a guideline is negligent or amounts to professional misconduct, is a question that should be answered by reference to the *Bolam* test. What we can say, though, is that a general practitioner should be very careful before departing from a guideline. He should have clearly thought out the reasons for doing this, and ideally, have discussed it with his colleagues. He should also note the reasons for his actions within the general practice record.

Inadequate communication

Several of the errors in the vincristine case can be categorised as communication errors. This is not surprising. Many errors in diagnosis and treatment can be traced back to inadequate communication. This may be between sequential general practitioners seeing the patient in the community, the Out of Hours service, the Accident & Emergency (A&E) department or poor li-aison after hospital discharge. In general practice it often comes down to the standard of the clinical notes (for the next clinician), the standard of the discharge summary or the communication between the general practitioner and, say, the district nurses or physiotherapists. In many cases of alleged delay in diagnosis the patient (with, for example, the subarachnoid haem-orrhage, pulmonary embolism or cervical cord compression) will have been seen by different general practitioners over a period of time, in A&E or by physiotherapists.

Communication can be achieved through the written or the spoken word. In the vincristine example, the doctor who was to administer the drugs and who took the afternoon off, should have done a formal face-to-face verbal handover with the doctor who was in charge of the ward that after-noon. Similarly, the loss of the child's medical records prevented the staff from comprehensively assessing the child's needs. Both these failings, one entailing verbal, the other written communication, denied others important information.

Reference

Department of Health (2000) *An Organisation with a Memory*, the report of an expert group on learning from adverse events in the NHS, chaired by the ChiefMedical Officer (2000). http://www.dh.gov.uk/en/Publication sand-statistics/Publications/PublicationsPolicyAndGuidance/DH_4065083.

Section 2: Causes of diagnostic errors in general practice and how they can be avoided

The huge majority of errors in general practice that result in litigation are alleged delays in diagnosis and referral. A significantly smaller proportion are due to incorrect prescribing or inadequate monitoring of treatment. An analysis of 1000 cases brought in the 1990s against general practitioners who were members of the Medical Protection Society found that 19% were due to medication or prescribing errors (Silk, 2000). We believe that that proportion of cases against general practitioners for prescribing errors has fallen due to computer generation of prescriptions and the increased number of claims relating to failure to diagnose.

How do general practitioners reach diagnoses?

In general practice a 'diagnosis' is more often a sort of junctional decision node rather than a histopathological entity with an objective existence. 'Mechanical low back pain' is distinguished from 'lumbar nerve root entrapment' because they are dealt with in a different way. Often the 'diagnosis' will effectively be that the condition is unlikely to be something serious – 'not DVT'.

The traditional model of diagnosis is one of initial collection of information with the history and examination. This is followed by deductive steps to reach the diagnosis. A more realistic model was formulated by Elstein *et al.* 25 years ago (Elstein and Schwarz, 2002). This model recognizes that the clinician often formulates a putative diagnosis very early on in the consultation – within the first couple of minutes. The doctor then recurrently, 'iteratively' tests this and a few other possibilities throughout the consultation (Norman *et al.*, 2009). The initial 'hypotheses' – rarely more than three or four possible diagnoses – are usually formulated before much data gathering has occurred. These are 'eyeball' first impressions. The choice of these initial possible diagnoses is strongly influenced by previous experience in the same situation. The first time a trainee general practitioner encounters the patient with vertigo or dizziness the doctor has rarely developed a diagnostic strategy. The 'apprenticeship' part of training usually involves developing strategies and heuristic models on which to hang the diagnostic pathway. Often, in simple examples, it may be possible to visualize the process as a flow diagram. An experienced diagnostician may only have to listen very carefully for sometime (allowing the patient time and room to express himself/herself) and then ask

Avoiding Errors in General Practice, First Edition. Kevin Barraclough, Jenny du Toit, Jeremy Budd, Joseph E. Raine, Kate Williams and Jonathan Bonser.
© 2013 John Wiley & Sons, Ltd. Published 2013 by John Wiley & Sons, Ltd.

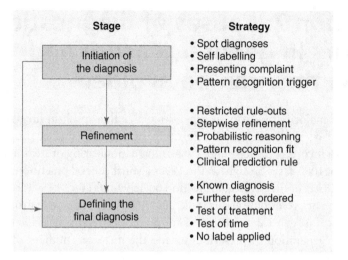

Figure 1.1 Stages and strategies in arriving at a diagnosis

two or three highly discriminating questions. The trainee may work out these template diagnostic models themselves or may observe them in colleagues or read them in articles or textbooks.

A study of 50 diagnostic consultations in general practice in the *BMJ* by Heneghan *et al.* (2009) concluded that the process of reaching a diagnosis could be modelled by three phases: initiation of the diagnosis (often very early in the consultation), refinement and then defining the diagnosis. The phases are illustrated in Figure 1.1.

Initiation of the diagnosis

The diagnosis may suggest itself as a 'spot diagnosis' as the patient walks through the door – Parkinson's, depression. The patient may have already 'self labelled' – 'I have trapped a nerve in my back', 'I have sinusitis'. Sometimes there may be a specific presenting complaint – headache. Often in general practice there is a panoply of symptoms and the general practitioner must decide which may indicate significant disease and which are unlikely to. Sometimes it is the recognition of a pattern when the individual features may be relatively subtle – the jaw ache with the headache (giant cell arteritis) or the urinary symptoms with the back pain (cauda equina syndrome).

Refinement

In the process of refinement of that initial impression it is important to 'second-guess' oneself. In many cases there are conditions that, though rare and of relatively low probability, are such that the consequences of missing them are too terrible to take the risk. It is worth sending 100 patients into hospital with a sudden onset severe headache to pick up one subarachnoid haemorrhage and avoid the catastrophic stroke in a 30 year old. Murtagh (1990) described this process as using the 'restricted rule out'.

In a differential diagnosis the condition at the top of the list should not be the most probable but the condition that you cannot afford to miss.

Once the initial impressions have been formed it is necessary to gather information that refines those possibilities – iteratively testing the various diagnoses. This often involves fitting the presentation to a pattern – this aching 70 year old who has difficulty getting out of a chair ('I'm getting old, doctor') may fit the pattern of polymyalgia rheumatic. However, it is often at this stage that errors are made – and we will discuss that below.

Often it is necessary, at some vague level of appreciation, to use probabilistic reasoning. A 20 year old with rectal bleeding is unlikely to have colorectal cancer.

In the past it was always extremely difficult to get information about how likely it was that a patient with a particular presentation had a given condition. Medical textbooks were encyclopaedias of diseases such as cryptogenic fibrosing alveolitis. The likelihood was loosely inferred from the incidence of the condition in the population.

In the last 20 years there is far more information about the predictive values of symptoms for particular conditions in particular age groups. Much of this data is from secondary care studies (A&E or specialist clinics). Since these populations are a highly selected group the results will usually not be applicable to general practice. However, increasingly there is primary care data that is obtained from interrogating anonymized computer data uploaded from primary care clinical systems, such as the General Practice Research Database (GPRD). The likelihood that a 65-year-old man with an unexplained haemoglobin of 11.5 g/dl and a low ferritin having colorectal cancer is about 6.5% (Hamilton *et al.*, 2008). The chances that a 70-year-old man with dysphagia has upper gastrointestinal cancer is about 9% (Jones *et al.*, 2007). The data is of course still relatively crude. The predictive value of a symptom is probably an order of magnitude higher if it is volunteered ('my food sticks, doctor') as compared with if it is elicited ('Do you ever notice that your food sticks? Well, yes, actually. A bit.')

There are now many useful repositories of such information. One of the first examples, starting in 1993, was the excellent series in the *Journal of the American Medical Association* (*JAMA*) called 'The Rational Clinical Examination' (Sackett, 1992). Now articles on evidence-based diagnosis are frequently published in the *British Medical Journal* (*BMJ*) and the *British Journal of General Practice* (*BJGP*). This information is usually couched in the language of Bayesian reasoning, and we will discuss that a little further below.

Clinical Prediction Rules (CPR) are increasingly a part of the diagnostic armament. Often they are developed and validated in secondary care (such as the Well's Scores for DVT and pulmonary embolism, or the Ottawa ankle rules). Secondary care CPRs have to be applied with caution in primary care because the populations are different, the initial likelihood of disease will be different (usually lower) and the clinical features that are discriminatory may be different (the absence of a central prostate sulcus on digital rectal examination is probably of relatively little discriminatory value to a urologist because few patients he sees will have a sulcus, whereas it probably is discriminatory for a general practitioner).

Sometimes the Clinical Prediction Rule may be problematic for the general practitioner if its specificity is poor, yet it finds its way into a national guidance document. An example is the 7-point check list for malignant melanoma that defines urgent referral criteria under the June 2005 NICE Guidelines for Suspected Cancer. The problem is that the specificity of the 7-point check list is only about 30–40% (Whited and Grichnik, 1998). Thus 60 or 70 out of 100 benign lesions in a pigmented lesion clinic will score 3 or more on the 7-point scale. A general practitioner cannot possibly urgently refer 60% of all the pigmented lesions she sees. Yet she may be criticized for not following guidelines if she fails to refer someone who turns out to have a malignant melanoma (see below for tips on how to avoid this problem).

Defining the final 'diagnosis'

As stated above, the 'diagnosis' may merely be a negation – this patient has not got cardiac chest pain. It may be a working strategy – this patient seems to have a peripheral rather than central cause for her vertigo so we will wait and see.

A relatively small number of patients in primary care can be given a confident diagnosis at first presentation. It is also important not to give diagnoses of misleading and spurious accuracy. Not all low back pain to one side of the midline is due to facet joint arthritis. Sometimes a misleading accurate diagnosis ('hemiplegic migraine') can be very misleading and harmful because the patient relies on the diagnosis and subsequent clinicians fail to reconsider this.

Sometimes it is necessary to try and refine the diagnosis with further tests, such as X-rays, blood tests or urinalysis. In these circumstances it is important that the general practitioner has some idea of the performance characteristics of the test. A normal chest X-ray does not exclude bronchial carcinoma in a 60-year-old smoker with haemoptysis. The sensitivity of spinal X-rays to detect vertebral metastases (for example, in a patient with a known history of prostate cancer and back pain) is only about 70%. It would be inappropriate (and a common source of diagnostic error) to rule the conditions out on the basis of a normal test result.

Sometimes a 'test of treatment' will help to clarify the diagnosis. If the chronic cough responds to a proton pump inhibitor it was likely to be due to gastro oesophageal reflux. However, this approach needs to be viewed with appropriate caution if there are potentially serious causes. It is no longer acceptable to make a diagnosis of angina on the basis of therapeutic response to a GTN spray.

Often in primary care it is necessary to allow some time for the diagnosis to become clear. The natural history of the condition determines the diagnosis. Acute diarrhoea is likely to be due to infective gastroenteritis if it settles over a week or 10 days. However, if the 'test of time' is to be used safely (for example, in the child with abdominal pain who does not seem to have appendicitis) then 'safety netting' is of critical importance. We will discuss this further below.

Quite commonly it is appropriate that no diagnostic label is applied. This may be unpopular with the patient, who will often welcome spurious diagnostic certainty. However, it may be the more honest and safer course of action. The diagnosis remains 'open' rather than 'closed' and both doctors and the patient acts accordingly.

If the patient has a long history of multiple symptoms that result in fruitless investigation it may be necessary to discuss with the patient the tradeoff between the risks of over investigation (and over diagnosis) and the risk of missing a diagnosis. If the reasoning is clear, logical, agreed with the patient and recorded, it may be possible to defend a failure in diagnosis in these circumstances. The question though of what constitutes consent on the part of the patient (for a decision, for example, not to be investigated or referred) will be discussed below.

Where do errors occur in diagnosis?

A type of 'taxonomy' of diagnostic errors can also be discerned from the diagnostic strategies outlined above by Heneghan *et al.* (2009). For convenience we will reproduce Figure 1.1 again.

Before discussing where on the diagram above the errors occur, it is worth considering the research into cognitive reasoning that has gone into this area. If we can identify common 'cognitive biases' that lead to error we can devise strategies to guard against them.

When diagnoses are missed it is usually assumed that it is due to inadequate data collection. Sometimes this may be the case. Often, however, this is not a consequence of sloppiness or inattention to detail; instead the critical bits of information are missed simply because the general practitioner did not think of the correct diagnosis. It never occurred to him that the patient, who may have had no obvious risk factors, may be breathless because of a pulmonary embolism. It was this failure, of even considering the diagnosis, which meant that he did not detect the swollen calf.

Quite often close analysis will show that the general practitioner has made one or more common cognitive errors.

General practitioners, like all clinicians, use cognitive heuristics that may lead to incorrect weighting of the evidence.

'Confirmation bias' leads to information gathering that will confirm rather than refute the diagnosis. If you think the 65-year-old man is hoarse because of gastro oesophageal reflux (GORD) then asking him about the presence of heartburn might appear to confirm the diagnosis. However, heartburn is so common in the population that its presence does not go anyway to excluding the diagnosis of bronchial carcinoma at the left carina. The confirmatory evidence is given too much weight. A more appropriate strategy would have been to refer for a chest X-ray and then referral for laryngoscopy, both to refute the (possibly more likely) diagnosis of GORD. Karl Popper's one millionth black swan refuted the general law ('all swans are white') that had been obtained by induction from the particular observations to the general law. A general practitioner should not carry out a million chest X-rays to detect one cancer (!) but the principle that confirmatory evidence is not necessarily discriminatory is often correct.

'Premature closure' is a common cause of diagnostic error in clinical negligence cases. The diagnosis of mechanical low back pain in a somatizing 50-year-old Asian lady may have been reasonable initially but, 3 months later when she was losing weight and sweating at night, the diagnosis needed to be rescrutinized. Unfortunately the general practitioner had already made up her mind that the woman was a depressed lady who 'catastrophized' her symptoms.

'Framing bias' is common in all areas of medicine. Once the CT scan shows the blood in the subarachnoid space the neurosurgical SHO elicits a perfect history of a subarachnoid haemorrhage, filling in the details not volunteered by the patient by direct questioning. The general practitioner may record a history that is absolutely typical for trigeminal neuralgia once he/she has decided that that is the diagnosis. There are many conditions in medicine in which the way the clinical data is 'framed' leads inexorably to a diagnosis – 'pleuritic chest pain', 'dry cough at night and on exertion'. In these circumstances it is important to be very careful about what information is volunteered by the patient and what (often confirmatory) data is elicited by direct questions – 'Do you cough a lot at night? Yes (but I also cough a lot during the day and sweat a lot at night).'

'Availability bias' is the process of giving too much weight to one's own past experience and easily recalled examples. Usually in primary care this leads to under diagnosis because serious conditions individually are relatively rare.

We will discuss simple strategies below that can help avoid falling into these 'cognitive traps'. However, first we give a few examples of the types of errors that can be anticipated from the real world structure of the diagnostic process imputed by Heneghan et al. (2009).

'Premature closure' on the spot diagnosis can lead to error unless the process is 'second guessed'. The patient may indeed be depressed, as seems to be the case, but this could be because of serious physical illness. The 'typical' left Bell's palsy may have weakness of grip in the left hand. Just because you have previously seen the 'pattern' of sudden onset of conjunctival oedema and periorbital swelling in a patient with allergic conjunctivitis does not mean that this person does not have a pre-septal orbital cellulitis. Beware of pattern recognition and 'availability bias'. The evidence is very clear that clinicians form their hypotheses very early on in the consultation. To be safe it is necessary to 'second guess' them at a later stage.

Patients' 'self labelling' is quite often correct. However, it is important not to put too much reliance on it. 'It's my old lumbago, doc' may turn out to have a vertebral metastasis, as occurs in nearly 1% of patients with back pain in primary care.

Equally, the presenting complain is quite frequently not the important part of the consultation. The throwaway remark about a 6-week history of loose stool with a bit of rectal bleeding in a 55-year-old woman consulting about marital problems is likely to be significant. It is important to realize that, even though the remark comes as she is walking through the door and you have already spent 20 minutes with her, it is crucial to deal safely with the problem. The initial event in many medico-legal cases is the throwaway remark as the patient heads for the door.

It is crucially important to use Murtagh's restricted rule out method. The first diagnosis on the list, so that you will actually consider it, is not the most likely but the one you must not miss. The difficulty with purely probabilistic reasoning is that the consequence of missing a diagnosis is often in inverse proportion to its probability. The febrile neonate probably has an upper respiratory tract infection but the consequences of delay of diagnosis of septicaemia can be catastrophic. The clinical suspicion and diagnosis of pulmonary embolism is very difficult. Many are missed. If you do not consider it first you will forget it and miss it.

How can we minimize the risks of these errors?

To finalize this section we suggest a few rules to help avoiding the cognitive errors that lead to misdiagnosis. These are the following 6 rules:

1. **Routinely second guess and consider the condition you cannot afford to miss**

   We can remind ourselves to routinely consider alternatives to our initial diagnosis – 'what can I not afford to miss? Am I sure that this person's red painful foot is cellulitis rather than critical ischaemia?'

2. **Seek data which would not fit with the hypothesis**

   We can specifically go after signs or symptoms that would be inconsistent with the diagnosis and suggest alternatives – such as facial weakness in Benign Positional Vertigo, or an explosive onset of headache in migraine.

3. **Reframe when recording**

   We can consciously re-examine the history as we write the notes. Do not merely record a history that fits in with our hypothesis – 'pulsating uni-lateral headache with nausea and visual aura'. Consider that the 'framing' may be misleading – the history of nausea was elicited in response to a direct question ('yes, a bit'), the term 'pulsating' was never used, the 'aura' was momentary visual 'greying'.

4. **Reconsider dissonant facts**

We can review and re-examine facts that don't quite fit. For example, perhaps this headache is far worse than any migraine the patient has ever had and she complains of slight neck stiffness. We can become more familiar with test accuracy: that an earlier, normal cervical smear does not exclude cervical cancer; a raised serum urate does not mean arthralgia is due to gout.

5. **Use time as a diagnostic test**

Appropriately timed follow-up may also allow the general practitioner to review the diagnosis and separate minor and time-limited conditions from potentially more serious problems. See the teenager with new onset of abdominal pain but no signs again the next day.

6. **Safety netting is an extremely powerful tool with which to cope with diagnostic uncertainty**

This is discussed in more detail in Part 1, Section 4. The mother looking after the febrile one year old should leave the consultation room with clear instructions about what to look for (mostly the 'Red and Amber' traffic lights in the May 2007 NICE guidance on Feverish illness in children (CG 47)), what she should do if these occur, contact details for Out of Hours if the practice is closed and follow up arrangements.

References and further reading

Del Mar C, Doust J, Glaszious P (2006) *Clinical Thinking: Evidence, Communication and Decision-Making.* Blackwell publishing (especially chapters 1 and 4).

Elstein A, Schwarz A (2002) Evidence base of clinical diagnosis: Clinical problem solving and diagnostic decision making: selective review of the cognitive literature. *BMJ* **324**: 729–32.

Hamilton W, Lancashire R, Sharp D, Peters TJ, Cheng KK, Marshall T (2008) The importance of anaemia in diagnosing colorectal cancer: a case-control study using electronic primary care records. *Br J Cancer* **98**: 323–7.

Heneghan C, Glasziou P, Thompson M, Rose P, Balla J, Lasserson D *et al.* (2009) Diagnostic strategies used in primary care. *BMJ* **338**: b946.

Jones R, Latinovic R, Charlton J, Gulliford MC (2007) Alarm symptoms in early diagnosis of cancer in primary care: cohort study using General Practice Research Database. *BMJ* **334**: 1040.

Murtagh J (1990) Common problems: a safe diagnostic strategy. *Australian Family Physician* **19**: 733–40.

NICE (2007) Feverish illness in children, CG 47; http://www.nice.org.uk/CG047

Norman G, Barraclough K, Dolovich L, Price D (2009) Iterative diagnosis. *BMJ* **339**: b3490.

Sackett DL (1992) A primer on the precison and accuracy of the clinical examination. *JAMA* **267**: 2638–44.

Silk N (2000) *An Analysis of 1000 Consecutive General Practice Negligence Claims.* MPS Casebook **8**.

Simel D, Rennie D (2009) *The Rational Clinical Examination: Evidence Based Clinical Diagnosis.* JAME.

Whited JD, Grichnik JM (1998) Does this patient have a mole or a melanoma? *JAMA* **279**: 696–701.

Section 3: Bayesian reasoning and avoiding diagnostic errors

Thomas Bayes was a very attractive eighteenth-century character who revolutionized reasoning in probability theory (he is buried in Bunhill Fields Cemetery in Moorgate, for those interested). He gave a mathematical structure to the notion that extra bits of information (in our case clinical bits of information) increase or decrease the probability of a particular diagnosis or outcome. Bayesian reasoning starts with the probability that a patient has a diagnosis before we know we know whether the patient has a particular clinical feature (say, fever) or a particular test result. This is the 'pre test probability'. We can then calculate a parameter known as a 'likelihood ratio' associated with the presence or absence of the clinical feature or test result. From the pre test probability and the likelihood ratio we can calculate the likelihood of disease after we know the additional clinical feature (say, whether the person has or has not a fever). This gives us the 'post test probability' of disease. This will be explained in more detail below.

Clinicians are 'natural Bayesians' (Gill *et al.*, 2005). We gather incremental bits of information in the consultation or with tests that refine the probability of a disease up or down.

In an ideal Bayesian world the patient would walk into the consulting room with a presenting complaint and the general practitioner would have a reasonable idea of the prior probability of a particular condition. It may be that the patient has acute onset of abdominal pain and the initial probability of it being due to acute appendicitis is about 1% (in fact that figure is from Emergency Department (ED) studies and the prior probability in general practice is likely to be much less). The general practitioner may then elicit the fact that the patient has right lower quadrant pain. This clinical feature has a positive likelihood ratio (LR+) of about 8 associated with it and, roughly, increases the probability to about 8% (Wagner *et al.*, 1996). If the pain started in the right lower quadrant and there was no migration of the pain this has a negative likelihood ratio (LR−) of about 0.5 and roughly halves the chance to about 4% (Wagner *et al.*, 1996). In this way the general practitioner may increase and decrease the probability of appendicitis by eliciting various features in the history and examination. At some stage the threshold would be reached where the probability was high enough to send the patient into hospital or low enough to give safety netting advice and/or arrange review and send them home (Pauker & Kassirer, 1980).

Avoiding Errors in General Practice, First Edition. Kevin Barraclough, Jenny du Toit,
Jeremy Budd, Joseph E. Raine, Kate Williams and Jonathan Bonser.
© 2013 John Wiley & Sons, Ltd. Published 2013 by John Wiley & Sons, Ltd.

In practice, this is a very unlikely scenario. There are many complicating factors. It is difficult to get good data about prior probability in primary care. The patient may have causes of acute abdominal pain other than acute appendicitis that are equally serious. Individual likelihood ratios are not necessarily independent of each other (which they would have to be to be applied sequentially).

However, there are aspects of the Bayesian model that are very useful in helping avoid the diagnostic errors outlined in the previous section and we will briefly illustrate a few of these here. The acronyms SpIN and SnOUT encapsulate useful rules for diagnosis (that are slightly counterintuitive). Tables of likelihood ratio do give us an idea of how useful bits of clinical information are in ruling a condition in or out. We will examine the 'Red Flags' in back pain as an example.

Generations of medical students have tried to remember the difference between sensitivity and specificity. They are, on the face of it, not very helpful or obvious metrics. However, when they are reformulated as likelihood ratios their meaning becomes a lot clearer.

In trying to remember sensitivity and specificity just remember two facts:
- **Sensitivity only deals with people with the disease.**
- **Specificity only deals with people without the disease.**

If a test or clinical feature in the history or examination has a sensitivity of 84% (right lower quadrant pain in acute appendicitis for example), then of 100 people with acute appendicitis, 84 will have right lower quadrant pain.

If a test or clinical feature has a specificity of 90% (right lower quadrant pain in acute appendicitis for example), then of 100 who have acute abdominal pain but do not have acute appendicitis, 90 will not have right lower quadrant pain. This is illustrated in Table 3.1.

We can also see from Table 3.1 that, if we just happened to have a population of 200 patients with acute abdominal pain, of whom 100 had acute appendicitis and 100 did not (a prevalence of 50%) then the probability that someone with right lower quadrant pain would have acute appendicitis (the positive predictive value of the sign) is $80/(80 + 10)$ or about 89%.

However, we can see that if the prevalence of acute appendicitis in the population being assessed is much lower, say 1%, the table looks quite different. Now there are roughly 100 times as many people without acute appendicitis as with acute appendicitis (the column on the right has 10 000 patients rather than 100 patients) (see Table 3.2).

Table 3.1

	Patients with acute appendicitis (100)	Patients without acute appendicitis (100)
Right lower quadrant pain	80	10
No right lower quadrant pain	20	90
	Sensitivity = 80/100	Specificity = 90/100

Table 3.2

	Patients with acute appendicitis (100)	Patients without acute appendicitis (10000)
Right lower quadrant pain	80	1000
No right lower quadrant pain	20	9000
	Sensitivity = 80/100	Specificity = 90/100

The sensitivity and specificity are the same (the reason why they are defined in such a counterintuitive way is that they are not dependent on prevalence). However, the positive predictive value of right lower quadrant pain is now only 80/(1000 + 80) or about 7%.

The positive predictive value of a clinical feature is highly dependent on the prior probability or the prevalence in the studied population. Most people with night sweats in an oncology unit will have lymphoma or opportunistic infections. Most people in general practice will not.

However, what we really want to know is how useful a clinical feature is for helping us avoid diagnostic errors. Likelihood ratios quantify the discriminatory value of a clinical feature.

The **positive likelihood ratio LR+** is the probability of a **positive** test result in patients with the disease, divided by the probability of a positive test result in patients without the disease. This is:

$$LR+ = \text{sensitivity}/(1\text{-specificity}).$$

The **negative likelihood ratio (LR−)** is the probability of a **negative** test result in patients with the disease, divided by the probability of a negative test result in patients without the disease. This is:

$$LR- = (1\text{-sensitivity})/\text{specificity}.$$

The full Bayesian equation is that:

Post-test odds of disease = the pre-test odd of disease x the likelihood ratio

where the odds of disease is (probability of disease/(1-probability of disease).

For our purposes we would very rarely use that equation. However, lists of positive and negative likelihood ratios are useful because they give us an idea of how good a particular feature is at helping us discriminate between those with the disease and those without.

A positive likelihood ratio (LR+) of 5 to 10 is very helpful. A value of 2 to 5 is quite helpful.

A negative likelihood ration (LR−) of 0.2 to 0.1 is very helpful. A value of 0.5 to 0.2 is quite helpful.

A LR close to 1 is useless.

We can illustrate this with figures taken from the article cited above on acute appendicitis. This is reproduced in Table 3.3.

Table 3.3 The sensitivity, specificity, positive and negative likelihood ratios for certain signs and symptoms of acute appendicitis.

Clinical feature	Sensitivity	Specificity	LR+	LR−
Right lower quadrant pain	0.81	0.53	1.8	0.4
Rigidity	0.27	0.83	1.6	0.9
Migration	0.64	0.82	3.6	0.4
Fever	0.67	0.79	3.2	0.4
Rebound tenderness	0.63	0.69	2.0	0.5
Guarding	0.74	0.57	1.7	0.5
Rectal tenderness	0.41	0.77	1.8	0.8
Anorexia	0.68	0.36	1.1	0.9
Nausea	0.58	0.37	0.9	1.1
Vomiting	0.51	0.45	0.9	1.1

We can see that, as we would expect, the presence or absence of right lower quadrant pain is quite helpful in discriminating between those with and without acute appendicitis. Nevertheless, relying on this feature alone will miss 19% of all cases of appendicitis. On the other hand the presence or absence nausea, vomiting or anorexia is largely useless. The LRs are too close to 1.

Likelihood ratios are also useful in defining the standard required of a general practitioner. 10 or 20 years ago it was accepted clinical wisdom that a digital rectal examination (DRE) was necessary in the assessment of acute abdominal pain ('put your finger in it or put your foot in it'). Many general practitioners were found in breach of duty for failing to carry out a DRE in a patient who subsequently was diagnosed with acute appendicitis. Studies such as those used to make the table above have shown that DRE is not generally useful in nonspecialist hands in making the diagnosis. The LR is close to 1 and it is now accepted that it should not be done in primary care as part of the assessment of someone with acute abdominal pain.

A last example of the usefulness of such tables is in the assessment of acute back pain. In the 1990s the Royal College of General Practitioners published a list of 'Red Flags' for people with back pain. These were clinical features that should cause general practitioners to be alerted to the possibility that the cause was not simple self limiting back pain. These features were as follows:
- Presentation under age 20 or onset over 55
- Nonmechanical pain
- Thoracic pain
- Past history – carcinoma, steroids, HIV
- Unwell, weight loss
- Widespread neurological symptoms or signs
- Structural deformity.

In cases that are brought against general practitioners for failure to diagnose or refer spinal cancer or infections the allegation is often that one or more of the first 3 'Red Flags' were present and mandated investigation. In fact studies

Table 3.4 The sensitivity, specificity, positive and negative likelihood ratios for certain signs and symptoms in the assessment of acute back pain.

	Sensitivity	Specificity	LR+	LR−
Age > 50	0.77	0.71	2.7	0.3
Nonmechanical pain	0.90	0.46	1.7	0.2
Thoracic pain	0.17	0.84	1.1	1.0
History of cancer	0.31	0.98	15.5	0.7

show the following 'performance characteristics' for 4 of the features listed (Deyo et al., 1992) (see Table 3.4).

What Table 3.4 shows clearly is that the presence of thoracic back pain (versus lumbar pain) is not useful as a discriminator. It is equally likely to occur in patients with or without cancer. A past history of cancer, on the other hand, is a powerful 'Red Flag' for cancer. It is absent in 98% of people with simple low back pain and present in 31% of those with vertebral metastases. Since plain X-rays only have a sensitivity of 70% for detecting cancer, one can infer that a patient with back pain and a history of cancer (particularly those cancers that tend to metastasize to bone such as breast, colon, prostate, lung, renal) probably needs an isotope bone scan.

Tables 3.3 and 3.4 also illustrate the usefulness of the acronyms SpIN (when a **sp**ecific test is **p**ositive, it rules the diagnosis **in**) and SnOUT (when a **s**e**n**sitive test is **n**egative, it rules the diagnosis **out**). In primary care the SpINs tend to be more plentiful and useful than the SnOUTs.

If we look again at Table 3.4 we see that the specificity of the history of cancer is 98%. That is to say that most people without vertebral metastases do not have that feature. If it is present it should ring alarm bells. If a clinical feature has a high specificity (Sp) but is Positive then the general practitioner should consider the possibility of serious disease firmly ruled IN.

SnOUTs are rarer in general practice. It is instructive to look at where errors are made because the doctor has considered that a negative finding on a test rules the condition out, when in fact it does not. Examples would be cervical smear tests or plain vertebral X-rays for metastases. The smear test has a sensitivity of about 80% for cervical cancer. That means that a general practitioner should not rely on a negative smear to rule out cancer because the sensitivity is too low. 20% of cases would be missed. It is not an adequate SnOUT. The same argument is true for plain X-rays looking for vertebral metastases.

An example of a SnOUT that is often quoted, and is useful if you are good with an ophthalmoscope, is the absence of retinal vein pulsations at the disc. This sign is present in all cases of raised intracranial pressure (sensitivity is 100%) (Jacks & Miller, 2003). Thus if retinal pulsations can be seen (the sign of absent pulsations is itself absent!) it rules the condition out. Thus, in a young person with a headache, if you can see retinal pulsations at the disc (and one often can in a young person) it rules the condition of raised intracranial pressure (from a tumour or benign intracranial hypertension) out.

References and further reading

Deyo RA, Rainville J, Kent DL (1992) What can the history and physical examination tell us about low back pain? *JAMA* **268**: 760–5.

Doust J (2009) Using probabilistic reasoning. *BMJ* **339**: b3823.

Gill CJ, Sabin L, Schmid CH (2005) Why clinicians are natural Bayesians. *BMJ* **330**: 1080–3.

Jacks AS, Miller NR (2003) Spontaneous retinal venous pulsation: aetiology and significance. *J Neurol Neurosurg Psychiatry* **74**: 7–9.

Pauker SG, Kassirer J (1980) The threshold approach to clinical decision making. *New England Journal of Medicine* **302**: 1109

Sackett DL (1992) A primer on the precision and accuracy of the clinical examination. *JAMA* **267**: 2638–44.

Tze-Wey Loong (2003) Understanding sensitivity and specificity with the right side of the brain. *BMJ* **327**: 716–19.

Wagner JM, McKinney WP, Carpenter JL (1996) Does this patient have appendicitis? *Journal of the American Medical Association* **276**: 1589–93.

Section 4: A potpourri of advice on avoiding errors

We have discussed what is involved in the diagnostic process and where the errors occur. We have discussed systematic methods of trying to overcome cognitive errors. We have discussed where Bayesian reasoning can inform our understanding of the clinical process of diagnosis. In Part 2 we will deal with the main purpose of the book – applying these principles to real life clinical scenarios.

However, we still need to cover a few more areas in which errors commonly occur such as clinical skills, communication problems, telephone consultations, the unexpectedly abnormal result, prescribing errors, drug monitoring errors, issues around consent, record keeping and the crucial aspect of 'safety netting'.

History and examination

Doctors, in general, are now far better at listening to patients then they were 20 years ago. When consultation techniques were first being analyzed and videotaped it became clear that doctors frequently interrupt a patient less than 30 seconds into their narrative. Clearly this is unwise because, in primary care, 90% of the diagnostic information is usually in the history. As the nineteenth-century clinician Sir William Osler who effectively created the modern clinical assessment said: 'Listen to the patient. He is telling you the diagnosis.'

The difficulty, of course, is that listening, like any observation, is not a passive business. It is necessary to concentrate and navigate what may be a blizzard of information. Patients vary greatly in their ability to describe their symptoms and concerns. The polysymptomatic middle-aged or elderly patient who is worried about everything is a particular concern. Many of the symptoms will be unlikely to signify serious disease but some will. It is difficult to walk the tightrope between over- and under-investigation in such patients. It is probably wise, if possible, to listen to their symptoms as it serves two purposes: first, it can be useful to look back some years later and see that the patient had those symptoms at that time too. Secondly, it potentially gives a more realistic picture of the difficulties of diagnosis if something is missed.

Examination skills have probably deteriorated since the time of Osler. One recent US book, Lisa Saunders' *Diagnosis* (Saunders, 2009) described

---

Avoiding Errors in General Practice, First Edition. Kevin Barraclough, Jenny du Toit, Jeremy Budd, Joseph E. Raine, Kate Williams and Jonathan Bonser.
© 2013 John Wiley & Sons, Ltd. Published 2013 by John Wiley & Sons, Ltd.

how newly qualified doctors rapidly give up on examination and 'just do the tests'. Neurological examinations seems to cause general practitioners particular problems. In fact, an enormous amount of information can be gained by simple examinations such as watching swallowing, watching the gait and manual dexterity. Many medico-legal cases are brought because the general practitioner has not felt for pedal pulses, checked visual acuity or pupillary reflexes, has not watched the patient walk or swallow, failed to feel the abdominal mass or visualize and feel the cervix in a woman with abnormal vaginal bleeding.

The telephone consultation

The telephone consultation has become a much commoner process since general practitioners in the UK gave up the requirement to do their own on call. Many patients contacting Out of Hours services are 'triaged' by telephone. These cases figure prominently in negligence.

A particular difficulty about the assessment of the patient Out of Hours or in any emergency setting is that the first role of the general practitioner is essentially to determine whether the patient is seriously ill and needs to be admitted to hospital. Much of the information that determines that assessment is usually visual. The patient looks unwell. He may be sweaty, have a poor colour or appear to have laboured breathing.

For the Court, and for good clinical practice, it is necessary to consider that the default standard of assessment required of a general practitioner is the standard that is possible when the patient is seen and examined. Anything less is a short cut which may or may not be justified. In a high profile case a few years ago a relatively young woman died of septicaemia after receiving telephone advice on five separate occasions over an Easter weekend. She was not seen or examined before her death.

When assessing the patient over the telephone it is necessary to try and envisage what is the range of possible scenarios on the other end of the phone. Are you confident that the patient with diarrhoea and vomiting is unlikely to be dehydrated (when did they last pass urine) or to have an acute surgical abdomen (if they have abdominal pain they need to be seen and examined)? How sure are you that the patient has a normal respiratory rate and colour? It is not enough that the patient does not request to be seen, or seems to be happy with advice. Usually in medico-legal cases concerning Out of Hours services there is a recording of the telephone consultation. Sometimes there are large gaps in the clinical information elicited. Sometimes the doctor gives advice before eliciting that the dizzy patient is on lithium, or that the vomiting patient is diabetic. Before hanging up on a telephone consultation it is necessary to ask yourself whether the clinical picture is absolutely clear, whether you can visualize that patient and have all the necessary information, whether the information from an abdominal examination or seeing the patient's breathing rate would be useful and whether all necessary 'safety netting' has been done.

Communication problems

In most medico-legal cases the patient has been seen by several doctors. Often there will be two or three general practitioners involved and an ED attendance. The patient may have seen the in house physiotherapist or district nurse. Sometimes one doctor may have requested a test and another sees the result. Each of these contacts is fraught with the difficulty that communication between the professionals may be unsatisfactory and key bits of information may be lost or not communicated. The physiotherapist may tell the patient to see the general practitioner because of urinary problems with back pain but the patient may fail to do so or may contact the general practitioner and not mention the detail that concerned the physiotherapist. Sometimes the problem is that the second general practitioner did not look back at the notes of the first and consequently missed a key clinical detail. He may not have checked the past medical history and missed that the patient had breast cancer 13 years earlier. The practice nurse may have noted that an ulcer that is failing to heal should be biopsied but this was never read or acted upon. In most cases there are several communication breakdowns.

To try and minimize this risk it is wise to always check the content of the past two or three consultation notes and have at least a cursory look at the past medical history and drug therapy before deciding on a management plan. Clear notes, which we will discuss in a moment, also make practice much safer.

When lack of knowledge plays a part

It is not possible for a general practitioner to know all that is necessary about all conditions and drugs. But in the modern information age it is very easy to look things up very quickly. A general practitioner should really be consulting the British National Formulary very regularly through the day. That episode of angio-oedema may be drug related. If you prescribe an angiotensin receptor blocker to a woman of child-bearing age it is necessary to be clear that they are teratogenic. There is extensive detailed and expert knowledge available on the web about conditions that general practitioners do not routinely look after, such as ulcerative colitis. It is always reasonable to look things up in a consultation, seek advice or revert to a patient later when you have found out more. It is often the over-confident general practitioner who ends up in court.

The unexpectedly abnormal result

A general practitioner will often see hundreds of separate results in a day. She may have only wanted a serum creatinine but she will get a sodium anyway. She may have requested an ALT and obtained a serum calcium anyway. A single request with ten numerical results has a nearly 50% statistical chance of having at least one result that is more than two standard deviations from the mean. Consequently, there will frequently be abnormal results. The sodium is only 129 mmol/l, the ALT is 86 UI/l, the platelets are 90.

Investigations can potentially lead to what Deyo describes as the 'cascade of technology' (Deyo, 2002). The routine ECG for a BUPA medical shows some inverted T waves, the echo is equivocal and the patient ends up having a coronary angiogram which is normal and a serious thigh haematoma.

However, failure to act on the unexpectedly abnormal result is a common cause of medico-legal cases. The raised ESR ends up being due to myeloma, the iron deficiency anaemia to cancer and high voltages on the ECG to aortic stenosis. The raised random glucose in 1997 is missed and leads to advanced retinopathy and nephropathy in 2009.

The general practitioner needs to adopt a careful and vigilant approach to abnormal results. Some can clearly be routinely ignored. The marginal abnormalities in subfractions of white cells, the sodium of 131 mmol/l. But most need to be treated with caution. A statistically freak result will normalize when it is repeated because of the statistical phenomenon of 'reversion to the mean'. Often that is all that is required. However, when a result is persistently abnormal it needs explaining. Often the explanation is relatively anodyne and requires no action. The patient with the sodium of 130 mmol/l is taking carbamazepine for epilepsy. But it is important to be aware that the abnormal result ticked as 'OK' may be a problem in the future. Even the instruction 'please repeat' may be a problem when it does not occur.

The standard of notes

General practice notes have historically been rather poor. When paediatric cases from the 1990s come to trial now (see the section on Limitations in Part 1, Section 1) it is necessary that the Court is aware that the average (and therefore *Bolam* defendable) standard of note keeping then would not be acceptable now.

Some general practitioners consider that detailed note taking is only necessary as part of medico-legally defensive practice. But this is not the case.

The standard of detail in consultation notes required by the General Medical Council is such that a subsequent clinician, reading the notes, would be able to reconstruct the clinical essentials of the consultation. In fact this standard is required for good clinical care, irrespective of any medico-legal considerations. The problems outlined in the section on communication between clinicians above are significantly amplified when the notes are poor. The patient is at greater risk of errors. It is also difficult to escape the conclusion that, although there are exceptions, poor notes often reflect poor clinical practice.

There are some basic details that are quite commonly omitted. It is good practice to record the duration of the symptom. 'Cough' is unacceptable. All that is required is 'cough 4/7' or whatever. Sometimes it is helpful to record key relevant negatives. The fact that the patient with a chronic cough has not lost weight is useful, particularly if she ends up having lymphoma. It is surprising how often general practitioners do not record the temperature, pulse and blood pressure in the febrile patient. It would not be possible to argue that a reasonable assessment was recorded when the patient subsequently dies of septicaemia.

It is necessary in the modern era to record some management plan and 'safety netting' advice unless it is truly self-evident from the consultation.

Some trainee general practitioners used to be embarrassed because they would come out of hospital practice and write long structured notes, only to see their senior colleagues writing one sentence.

Although brevity is to be valued, it is good practice to keep some semblance of the old SOAP (Subject, Object, Assessment, Plan), or 'history, examination, diagnosis, plan' structure and to second guess yourself. Ask yourself whether a colleague could work out from your notes the essential details of the consultation.

Drug errors or prescribing errors

It does appear that in general practice, because of the computerized prescribing systems, errors in doses are less common, though it is clearly more of a risk with paediatric dosing.

The more common allegations are inappropriate prescribing, inappropriate monitoring or failing to recognize drug side effects. Prolonged benzodiazepine prescribing remains a common cause of litigation. Inadequate monitoring of drugs such as azathioprine, lithium, phenytoin or prednisolone are relatively common causes of litigation.

Consent

The aspect of consent that features sometimes in negligence cases against general practitioners is when the patient initially decides not to be referred into hospital with an acute medical condition. The general practitioner may record 'patient not keen on admission'. The patient then dies from a pulmonary embolism.

If a competent general practitioner would have sought to admit the patient, the patient's decision not to go to hospital only absolves the general practitioner if it was a fully informed decision. The general practitioner needs to have explained all *the material risks* in making such a decision. The risks it is necessary to explain are those that a reasonable general practitioner would advise to their patient. In other words, the standard is based on the *Bolam* test. Usually it would be necessary to explain any diagnostic uncertainty ('I think you have a chest infection but it may be a pulmonary embolism') and the range of possible outcomes ('if you do not go into hospital you may die').

Sometimes an elderly patient, or a patient with terminal disease, may elect not to be admitted into hospital. But 'patient not keen on admission' is only likely to be a defence if the patient made a fully informed decision.

Consent features are more straightforward in cases about minor procedures carried out in general practice. Was the young woman informed of the risk of keloid if she had the lesion excised from the necklace area on her chest? Again, the duty is to inform of all material risks that might inform a reasonable person's decision.

If a general practitioner handles the above examples with insufficient care, he may find himself facing a negligence claim. The last issue of consent we will cover is more likely to arise in a complaint against a general practitioner rather than a negligence case. It is the question of the competence of a child or an adult with diminished capacity to consent to treatment.

It is important to understand that the test is whether the person has the capacity to consent to *that particular decision*. It is not a global assessment of whether the patient has the capacity to make any decision. A person may have the capacity to consent to have a minor operation to remove a mole, but may not have the capacity to make a complicated life and death decision about whether to be admitted into hospital or not.

A person is competent, if he can:
- understand and retain information pertinent to the decision about his care, i.e. the nature, purpose and possible consequences of the proposed investigations or treatment, as well as the consequences of not having treatment;
- use this information to consider whether or not he should consent to the intervention offered;
- communicate his/her wishes.

Children aged 16 and over are presumed to have the same capacity as an adult to consent to medical treatment (Family Law Reform Act, 1969).

Except in emergencies, the consent of a parent or, more accurately, someone with parental responsibility will be required for children under 16 who lack the capacity to understand the nature of the treatment being offered.

A child under the age of 16 may have capacity, provided she is capable of understanding the nature of the proposed course of treatment and is capable of expressing that wish. Such a child is referred to as *Fraser* (or *Gillick*. The two terms can be used interchangeably) competent. There is no fixed age at which a child becomes *Fraser* competent. It depends on the maturity of each individual child. Usually, the *Fraser* test will cause few difficulties, as both parent and child will agree on the treatment and be involved in the decision-making process. The problem typically arises when a young girl turns up at the surgery asking for contraception or a termination of pregnancy, determined to keep her treatment or condition from her parents. Then the doctor will have to carefully assess the capacity of this child, to determine whether she is competent to understand.

Confidentiality

'Whatever I see or hear, professionally or privately, which ought not to be divulged, I will keep secret and tell no one.' The words are those of Hippocrates. They form part of his oath and are still an important article of the doctor/patient relationship. Hippocrates simply gives voice to the fact that a full history is an essential requirement for diagnosis and treatment and the patient must feel able to tell his doctor everything relevant to his condition, even the most embarrassing and personal details, without fear that those details will be divulged to others. Updating the words of Hippocrates and putting them in legal terms, a doctor owes a duty of confidence regarding information about his patient or others acquired in his capacity as a doctor. This duty applies whether the information comes from other people or from the patient himself.

If a doctor breaches this duty of confidence, then he could be sued for damages, but more likely he will be reported to the GMC. As far as it affects clinicians, the law concerning confidentiality is fashioned from a number of different sources. Primarily, there is the common law duty of confidence (constructed from court judgements). In the last few decades, this has been supplemented by a number of Acts of Parliament: namely, The Access to Health Records Act (1990), The Data Protection Act (1998) and The Human Rights Act (1998). These different elements combine to create a more or less coherent whole. What we have set out below represents a basic outline of this legal framework.

Starting with the basics, a doctor can disclose information to others, if he has the patient's consent. But consent can be implied. Most patients understand that a doctor will share information about them with other members of the health team. In other words, the doctor can assume that he has the patient's implied consent to do this.

This may seem obvious, but a doctor should, where appropriate, consider just how far this implied consent extends for any given course of treatment. It may not extend to highly personal details about the patient that he has learned in treating some other, previous illness. The doctor should consider what information it is necessary to disclose to other members of the healthcare team, when treating the child. If he discloses information of a highly personal nature, then he should make it clear that the information is disclosed to them in confidence. He should also tell the patient that the information has been shared with other members of the team.

Data Protection Act, 1998

Generally speaking, patients seek disclosure of their records under the Data Protection Act. It is most frequently 'used' for this purpose. However, disclosure of records represents only a small part of its purpose.

The Act requires every practice to have in place a number of protocols to safeguard the confidentiality of patient information. For example, the physical paper records should be carefully stored in a secure environment. Any electronic data (e.g. radiographs) should be protected with access only allowed to those with passwords.

Disclosure without consent

There are a number of circumstances in which a doctor can legitimately disclose patient information to another without the consent of the patient:

- *Abuse or neglect*: Where the doctor believes that a child may be the victim of abuse or neglect and he is unable to give or withhold consent for disclosure, then the child's health is of paramount importance and he may disclose his belief to an appropriate, responsible person.
- *Statutory obligation*: A doctor is required to notify the appropriate authorities, if he attends upon someone suffering from an infectious disease or someone who is known or suspected to be addicted to controlled drugs.
- *Public interest*: A doctor may disclose patient information, if he believes that the patient presents a real risk of danger or serious harm to the public.
- *When ordered by the court to do so*: A doctor should not assume that simply because a lawyer or some figure of authority, such as a police officer, asks for disclosure of the patient's records, they are entitled to see the medical records. He should only disclose the records, if the patient has consented or the court has ordered disclosure.

Caldicott Guardians

Each health service body, including GP practices, should employ a Caldicott Guardian. His role is to ensure that patient information is dealt with in an appropriate fashion and that there are systems in place to ensure that all doctors generally respect the duty of confidentiality that exists between them and the patients that they serve. Therefore, he should be a first port of call, if an issue arises concerning the use of confidential information.

Conditions that are 'frequent flyers' in negligence cases

There are some conditions that are very over-represented in medical negligence cases. It is worth keeping them at the back of your mind when assessing patients. 'Could this patient have . . . ?' Here are a few:

- *Subarachnoid haemorrhage.* Always ask about the onset of the headache. Was it abrupt? Bear in mind that the headache can take minutes to reach full severity in 50% of cases. Beware the headache at the back of the neck.

- *Pulmonary embolism.* 22% do not have features of pulmonary infarction or collapse and present with breathlessness alone. Always consider it with unexplained breathlessness.
- *Cauda equina syndrome.* Very rare in normal practice and very common in medico-legal cases. Always ask about urinary symptoms and abnormal sensation in the saddle area. Ideally, warn about the significance of the same.
- *Acute appendicitis.* Be aware that a significant proportion do not present in the classical way. There may be urinary symptoms or diarrhoea that misleads the general practitioner. Signs of right lower quadrant tenderness may be absent if the appendix is retrocaecal.
- *Ischaemic feet.* Beware of 'gout' or 'cellulitis' in a pulseless foot. The red painful foot may be critically ischaemic. Always check for pulses, with a Doppler if impalpable. It is good practice to do an ABPI (Ankle Brachial Pressure Index), especially if there is an ulcer. Refer diabetics with an ulcer to a 'multi-disciplinary diabetic foot team' within 24 hours (required under NICE, 2004).
- *Malignant melanoma.* With pigmented lesions, even if they appear benign, measure them and see them again in 6 weeks if there is an uncertain history of possible change.
- *Breast cancer.* Re examine in 6 weeks if you cannot feel the lump the patient felt. Be aware that even a competent clinical breast examination misses many cancers that are less than 2 cm in diameter.
- *Colorectal cancer.* Be aware of the significance of asymptomatic mild, iron deficiency anaemia, rectal bleeding and a change in bowel habit to loose stools. Always do a digital rectal examination and feel the abdomen.
- *Cervical cancer.* A young woman on the pill may have breakthrough bleeding, but once it persists despite a pill change the cervix needs examining. A recent normal smear is not a SnOUT.
- *Diabetic ketoacidosis.* Always check the urine for ketones in an unwell patient with Type 1 diabetes. Admit if more than 1 + ketones.
- *Achilles tendon rupture.* With the ankle injury ask about any 'snap', check they can stand on tip toe and do the 'calf squeeze test'.
- *Septicaemia.* Always measure and record a temperature, pulse and blood pressure in a febrile patient.
- *The unexpectedly abnormal result.* The default is usually to repeat it.

Safety netting

The last issue in this section is of crucial importance in general practice.

The general practitioner is in the unenviable task of making assessments and decisions in an environment when there is usually considerable diagnostic uncertainty and the patient is not supervised as they would be in hospital.

It is neither practical nor good medicine to investigate all patients to the degree that they will be investigated in secondary care. An important part of the role of the general practitioner is to protect the patient against the iatrogenic harm that comes about if the patient is unnecessarily exposed to a 'cascade' of medical technology inherent in searching for an elusive diagnosis.

In addition, the illness may evolve in an unpredictable way. A two year old with an unremarkable upper respiratory tract infection may abruptly deteriorate. Most adults with community acquired pneumonia can be managed at home, but one may unexpectedly develop septicaemia or respiratory failure. The teenager with the abdominal pain may have no features of acute appendicitis when assessed but may then start vomiting and developing right lower quadrant peritonism.

The general practitioner's powerful magic weapon is 'safety netting'.

Twenty years ago the safety net involved saying 'come back if you don't get better' and recording 'SOS'. Safety netting is now a more evolved beast. It extends from, at one end, the advice above. Most minor illness in primary care is self-limiting and the patient does not routinely need to be reviewed. If the patient's course deviates from the expected natural history (they still have diarrhoea in 7 days) then they need review but otherwise they do not.

A more elaborate form of safety netting is the planned review, together with advice about what to do if the situation deteriorates in the interim. 'You have no signs of acute appendicitis now but I would like to see you again tomorrow after morning surgery. If things get worse overnight then you should call the Out of Hours service and this is the number.'

A more elaborate form still is to specify the symptoms that should prompt the patient to seek review. Most patients with acute low back pain will not appreciate the significance of having difficulty passing urine or abnormal sensation in the saddle area. Warning them of the significance of this may mean that they seek help at an early stage rather than having a complete cauda equina syndrome and having a neuropathic bladder for 48 hours before seeking advice.

The gold standard is a written advice sheet. 'Your febrile 2 year old does not seem to have any serious illness at the moment but very rarely a child can become very unwell very quickly. If you are at all concerned ring this number. We would be particularly concerned about fast breathing, unreasonable distress, unrousable drowsiness, poor fluid intake, wet nappies spaced by more than 4 hours, cold or mottled hands or feet or a rash that doesn't blanch. This sheet outlines the things that would worry us and instructions of what to do.'

It would not be reasonable to be critical of a general practitioner who carried out a careful assessment and safety netted carefully, merely because the child later developed signs of a serious illness. Documenting advice given is clearly also good practice.

Safety netting is a very powerful weapon with which to deal safely with uncertainty in general practice.

References and further reading

Almond S, Mant D, Thompson M (2009) Diagnostic safety-netting. *British Journal of General Practice* **59**: 872–4.

Deyo RA (2002) Cascade effects of medical technology. *Annual Review of Public Health* **23**: 23–44.

General Medical Council (2008) *Consent Guidance: Patients and Doctors Making Decisions Together.* GMC.

NICE (2004) NICE guideline to Type 2 diabetes – footcare. CG10.

Saunders L (2009) *Diagnosis: Dispatches from the Frontlines of Medical Mysteries.* Icon Books Ltd.

PART 2

Clinical cases

Introduction

Having set the scene with a general discussion of error and medico-legal theory, we now come to the backbone of our book: the case studies. We have chosen 40 cases which are based on actual scenarios but which have been anonymized and altered to preserve confidentiality and to maximize the educational messages of the case. In addition to a medical and legal comment, at various points in the description of a case, we ask direct questions that are designed to engage the reader in the case and to get them to think about how they would respond if they were in that situation. The case studies are rounded off with key learning points.

The medical comment is provided in the section entitled 'Expert Opinion'. In the Legal Comment section, reference is often made to the 'instructed expert'. This instructed expert refers to the expert that the defendant general practitioner or the claimant may instruct as part of the litigation process. It will be no surprise that experts may differ in their opinions. As much as it is a science, medicine is also an art. There is often room for argument over the finer points of a case. But that does not obviate the general conclusions that we draw, or the benefits that can be gained from the reading of our case studies.

They are here to make the reader think and if we succeed in doing that, then we will already have gone some way in achieving our aim of reducing the number of clinical errors.

Avoiding Errors in General Practice, First Edition. Kevin Barraclough, Jenny du Toit, Jeremy Budd, Joseph E. Raine, Kate Williams and Jonathan Bonser.
© 2013 John Wiley & Sons, Ltd. Published 2013 by John Wiley & Sons, Ltd.

Case 1 A man with iron deficiency

Jeff is a 53-year-old man who returned from a two-week holiday visiting family in Kenya with symptoms of a febrile illness. He had taken antimalarials but was concerned about malaria. He consults Dr Wallace. She finds that he is apyrexial and looks well but she requests a full blood count and films for malarial parasites. The films are negative for parasites. The FBC shows a haemoglobin of 12.3 g/dL and a MCV of 67 fL (normal ranges > 13.5 g/dL and 70 to 100 fL). The results are filed.

What would you have done with the results?

Four months later Jeff consults another of GP in the practice, Dr Rennie, with a two-week history of a dry cough and fatigue. Examination is unremarkable, urinalysis and TFTs are normal but the Hb is 10.7 g/dL with a MCV of 66 fL. Dr Rennie diagnoses an iron deficiency anaemia, requests haematinics, starts Jeff on ferrous sulphate and requests a repeat blood test in two months. The serum ferritin is 10 mcg/l. Dr Rennie suggests doing three faecal occult bloods. Two are done and are negative. Two months later the repeat FBC result comes back to the ST2 trainee, Dr Bordley. The man's haemoglobin is now 13.6 g/dL with a MCV of 70 fL.

What would you do now? What is your differential diagnosis?

Dr Bordley asks the receptionists to contact Jeff for a routine appointment. Unfortunately Jeff fails to make an appointment as requested.

Six months later Jeff consults Dr Rennie again, this time with fatigue. He is clinically anaemic. He stopped taking the ferrous sulphate some months earlier. Abdominal examination suggests a right lower quadrant abdominal mass. A FBC shows a Hb of 9.1 g/dL with an MCV of 66 fL. Dr Rennie refers Jeff urgently to a consultant gastroenterologist and a colonoscopy shows

a circumferential, stenosing caecal carcinoma. He undergoes a right hemicolectomy and the cancer is staged as Dukes C1.

Jeff sues the three general practitioners on the premise that his iron deficiency anaemia should have been investigated one year earlier and that this would have led to an earlier diagnosis of the cancer with a better prognosis.

Expert opinion

As with many medico-legal cases there are often a number of errors which compound the delay in diagnosis. Iron deficiency in a man in the developed world is rarely due to dietary deficiency (Goddard *et al.*, 2005). In contrast, menstruating women can easily tip into a negative iron balance because of a significant monthly loss with menstruation. Anaemia indicates significant iron deficiency following exhaustion of the marrow stores. Iron deficiency anaemia in a man is rare and always needs investigating. It must never be assumed to be dietary because such an assumption is unsafe and rarely true.

Since July 2000 the UK 'Two Week Rule' referral guidelines have recommended urgent referral for men with an iron deficiency anaemia of less than 11 g/dL in a man and 10 g/dL in a non menstruating woman (NHS Executive, 2000). However, the 2005 British Society of Gastroenterology (BSG) guidance is to refer for investigation all men and women with an unexplained iron deficiency anaemia of any degree (Goddard *et al.*, 2005). The likely causes are occult blood loss from a carcinoma or peptic ulceration (particularly with NSAIDs) or malabsorption due to, for example, Coeliac's disease. Most right-sided colorectal cancers present with an isolated iron deficiency. Right-sided colorectal cancers often do not cause the characteristic alteration in bowel habit (to loose, frequent stools) that occurs with left-sided cancers. Cancers proximal to the splenic flexure will also not produce rectal bleeding.

One study of 695 patients with iron deficiency anaemia referred under the BSG guidance found

Avoiding Errors in General Practice, First Edition. Kevin Barraclough, Jenny du Toit, Jeremy Budd, Joseph E. Raine, Kate Williams and Jonathan Bonser.
© 2013 John Wiley & Sons, Ltd. Published 2013 by John Wiley & Sons, Ltd.

colorectal cancer in 6.4% (James *et al.*, 2005). A second study of 431 patients with a haemoglobin below 12 g/dL in men and 11 g/dL in women found 7.4% had colorectal cancer (Logan *et al.*, 2002). Another case-controlled study using a retrospective analysis of primary care computerized records identified 6442 patients with colorectal cancer and 45 066 controls. For men with an iron deficiency anaemia the positive predictive value of iron deficiency anaemia for colorectal cancer was 13.3% (Hamilton *et al.*, 2008).

The request for faecal occult bloods is an example of a clinician not understanding the performance characteristics (sensitivity and specificity) and therefore significance of a requested test. The test was incorrectly being requested as a 'rule out test' – if the FOBs were negative the GP would consider that occult bleeding had been 'ruled out'. However, the sensitivity of the test was too low to be a 'rule out test'. The sensitivity of three FOBs is only 50% to 90% for colorectal cancer (Hewitson *et al.*, 2007). Many people with colorectal cancer will still have three negative tests. To rule out a diagnosis, the test has to have a high sensitivity (like a barium enema) and be negative. The acronym is SnOUT – high sensitivity negative test rules it out.

The initial assessing GP, Dr Wallace, should have recognized that iron deficiency anaemia in a man, even if mild, requires confirming with a serum ferritin level and then investigating if it is confirmed. Jeff would not have met the criteria for an urgent 'Two Week Rule' referral (the Hb needs to be below 11 g/dL) but should have been referred non-urgently for specialist gastroenterological opinion.

The second GP Dr Rennie correctly requested a repeat full blood count and a serum ferritin but should then have referred the patient urgently to see why he had an iron deficiency anaemia. The faecal occult blood tests were inappropriate. They are colorectal cancer screening tests for an asymptomatic population.

The ST2 doctor Dr Bordley should have recognized that there was a high probability that Jeff had serious gastro intestinal disease (cancer or an ulcer) and ensured that he was seen rather than have merely delegated contacting the man to a receptionist.

 ## Legal comment

Expert comment confirms that Dr Wallace ought to have also carried out a serum ferritin test to rule out iron deficiency anaemia, an indicator of colorectal cancer. Although Jeff did not meet the criteria for an urgent two-week referral he ought to have been referred

non-urgently for specialist gastroenterological opinion because of the low haemoglobin results.

Four months later Jeff returned to his GP practice with a dry cough and fatigue and saw Dr Rennie. Although Dr Rennie diagnosed iron deficiency anaemia she failed to refer Jeff for investigation of the unexplained iron deficiency.

The mistakes continued when the ST2 Trainee Dr Bordley failed to recognize the high probability that Jeff had serious gastro intestinal disease from the results of the repeat FBC.

Six months later Jeff consulted Dr Rennie again when she found a right-sided abdominal mass on examination and appropriately referred Jeff to a consultant gastroenterologist.

All three doctors failed to consider any differential diagnoses. They appeared not to be aware of BSG guidance or the Two Week Rule guidance. Communication between all three doctors about Jeff's unexplained anaemia appears to have been poor. A breach of duty by the GPs seems clear. The next question is what the results of that breach were. It is fortunate that the cancer seems to be confined to the right side of the colon and has not spread beyond it. Had Jeff been properly diagnosed with iron deficiency anaemia and appropriately referred to a specialist gastroenterologist at the outset, his prognosis may not have been any different. (He may still have required surgery.) If expert opinion confirms that it is unlikely that the prognosis would have been any different had the cancer been identified earlier, then Jeff could expect to be awarded damages for approximately one year's pain and suffering with contributions being made by all three doctors.

 ## Key learning points

Specific to the case
• Iron deficiency anaemia in men should never be assumed to be dietary as this is unlikely and an unsafe assumption.
• Approximately 10% of men with unexplained iron deficiency anaemia will have colorectal cancer, often of the caecum.

General points
• It is important to know the performance characteristics of a test before relying on it to 'rule in' or 'rule out' a diagnosis.
• It is only sensible to 'rule out' a condition if the test has a high sensitivity and is negative – SnOUT.

References and further reading

Goddard AF, James MW, McIntyre AS, Scott BB (2005) Guidelines for the management of iron deficiency anaemia. British Society of Gastroenterology.

Hamilton W, Lancashire R, Sharp D, Peters TJ, Cheng KK, Marshall T (2008) The importance of anaemia in diagnosing colorectal cancer: a case-control study using electronic primary care records. *Br J Cancer* **98**: 323–7.

Hewitson P, Glasziou P, Irwig L, Towler B, Watson E (2007) Screening for colorectal cancer using the faecal occult blood test, Hemoccult. Wiley Online Library. DOI: 10.1002/14651858.CD001216.pub2

James MW, Chen CM, Goddard WP, Scott BB (2005) Risk factors for gastrointestinal malignancy in patients with iron deficiency anaemia. *European Journal of Gastroneterology and Hepatology* **17**: 1197–1203.

Logan E, Yates J, Steward R, Fielding K, Kendrick D (2002) Investigation and management of iron deficiency anaemia in general practice: a cluster randomised controlled trail of a simple management prompt. *Postgraduate Medical Journal* **78**: 533–7.

NHS Executive (2000) *Referral Guidelines for Suspected Cancer*, 19–20. London, Department of Health.

Case 2 When is a headache abrupt?

Hannah was 36 when she presented to an Out of Hours general practitioner, Dr Walmesley, situated in an emergency department (ED). She had a headache. She was a known migraine sufferer but had not suffered from migraine for a couple of years and felt that this was the worst attack she had suffered for many years and that her routine analgaesia was inadequate. She stated that four years earlier she had been referred to a specialist with episodes of vertigo associated with headache and the diagnosis had been migraine. Her current headache had come on 6 hours earlier. It was initially in the neck and back of the head and had progressively worsened over 10–15 minutes to being very severe. She had vomited once. On examination she was afebrile with no neck stiffness and no abnormalities other than mild photophobia on retinal examination. Dr Walmesley diagnosed migraine and prescribed strong opiates and an anti-emetic.

What would you have done?

Two days later the woman consulted her own general practitioner Dr Palmer. She told the doctor that she had been to hospital two days earlier and that the hospital had diagnosed migraine but that the painkillers were only relieving the headache for a couple of hours. She had a minor degree of neck ache and stiffness. There was no abnormality on examination and Dr Palmer suggested the use of a tryptan.

What would you do now? What is your differential diagnosis?

Ten days later Hannah was found dead in bed. A post-mortem revealed a large recent subarachnoid haemorrhage (SAH) originating from a 25 mm basilar artery Berry aneurysm. Hannah's family sued the general practitioners for negligently making a diagnosis of migraine. It was argued that a competent general practitioner

would have admitted her for urgent investigation, that an MRI would have demonstrated the Berry aneurysm and that it would have been treated with an endovascular coil.

Do you think their claim will succeed?

 ## Expert opinion

The suspicion and referral of patients suspected of having a SAH or 'warning bleeds' present a very significant problem for general practitioners and ED staff. Few general practitioners would fail to suspect a SAH in a patient with the typical presentation of an abrupt onset of a very severe occipital headache (thunderclap headache).

However, case studies indicate that abrupt onset of a headache may not occur in up to 50% of cases (Linn *et al.*, 1994). The time from onset to peak severity maybe several minutes (Linn *et al.*, 1998). This may explain why case studies of SAH find initial rates of misdiagnosis of between 23% and 51%.[3] The patients who are misdiagnosed tend to be less unwell, usually with no transient loss of consciousness and have no neurological signs. The commonest incorrect diagnosis is migraine (21% of misdiagnoses).

Even if an explosive headache is the only presenting symptom only 10% will have SAH (Edlow & Caplan, 2000). Nevertheless, it is obviously worth referring and investigating 10 patients (or even 100) to detect one SAH at an early stage. The more difficult question is whether to refer all patients with the 'worst headache ever' even if it comes on over several minutes. One US study found that 20 out of 107 patients presenting to an ED department with the 'worst ever' headache had SAH (Morgenstern *et al.*, 1998). However, one community study found that 9.1% of the population reported at least one 'almost unbearable' headache in the previous year (Newland *et al.*, 1978). Potentially, the whole

Avoiding Errors in General Practice, First Edition. Kevin Barraclough, Jenny du Toit, Jeremy Budd,
Joseph E. Raine, Kate Williams and Jonathan Bonser.
© 2013 John Wiley & Sons, Ltd. Published 2013 by John Wiley & Sons, Ltd.

population of headache sufferers will have their 'worst ever headache' at some stage. While the presence of neck stiffness makes the diagnosis more likely one unpublished study from Durham found neck stiffness was absent in 64% of cases of SAH. Nuchal rigidity may take 3 to 12 hours to develop, and maybe absent in small bleeds.

Duration of headache can be helpful in excluding SAH. It is generally accepted that the headache from a SAH usually lasts days and certainly does not last less than an hour (Davenport, 2002).

The conclusion of the studies is that clinical suspicion of a SAH needs to be set at a low level because up to half the cases may not present with a typical thunderclap headache. Nevertheless, close questioning about the onset of a headache is critical to the assessment of any new headache and details about onset should be recorded. Brief duration headaches that resolve are not due to SAH but general practitioners should have a low threshold for urgently referring sudden onset headaches or 'first and worst' headaches even if the onset is over a few minutes and there are no neurological signs such as nuchal rigidity.

Dr Walmesley should have recognized that SAH was a significant possibility (the chance of SAH was probably about 1 in 10) and admitted Hannah urgently to hospital for a CT head scan and a lumbar puncture. The second general practitioner Dr Palmer should have retaken the crucial history about the onset of the symptoms and realized that a SAH may have been missed and again admitted her urgently. Dr Palmer should not have been reassured by the earlier negative assessment 'in hospital'.

 Legal comment

The duty of a GP is to act in accordance with a responsible body of medical opinion skilled in that particular field. The expert in this case believes that both Dr Walmesley and Dr Palmer have failed to do so. He says they should both have recognized the possibility of SAH and arranged for further investigations.

However, a lawyer acting for either of those two doctors may wish to explore whether there is another responsible body of medical opinion which takes a different view. Maybe it could be argued for Dr Walmesley that the lack of neurological symptoms and the history of a gradual progression of the headache made it reasonable for him to diagnose migraine at the first consultation? (No doubt it will be more difficult for an expert to argue this for Dr Palmer who saw Hannah two days later when

she had a persistent headache and some neck ache and stiffness.)

The lawyers for the doctors will also want to explore the consequences of the failure to refer Hannah for investigation. Was it more likely than not that Hannah could have been saved if referred for a CT scan? If so, then Hannah's family will have a valid claim for bereavement damages of £11 800. The administrators of her estate could sue for the pain and suffering she endured before her death, due to the GP's negligence. If Hannah has children, they will have a potentially substantial claim as her dependents for the loss of care and support from their mother during their childhood. The family will also be entitled to compensation representing her financial contribution to the household.

 Key learning points

Specific to the case
- The headache in a SAH may take several minutes to reach peak severity.
- The history of the onset is critical to making the diagnosis.
- There may be no physical signs.
- Consider SAH in all cases of sudden onset severe headache and the 'first and worst' headache that lasts more than an hour.

General points
- General practitioners should not rely on a diagnosis of a headache made by the clinician who saw the patient first. Even in hospital the assessing doctor may have been inexperienced. Always retake the history, particularly of the onset.

References and further reading

Davenport R (2002) Acute headaches in the emergency department. *J Neurol Neurosurg Psychiatry* **72**: 33ii–37.

Edlow JA, Caplan LR (2000) Avoiding pitfalls in the diagnosis of subarachnoid hemorrhage. *N Engl J Med* **342**: 29–36.

Hankey GJ, Nelson MR (2009) Easily missed: Subarachnoid haemorrhage. *BMJ* **339**: 569–70.

Linn FHH, Wijdicks EFM, van Gijn J, Weerdesteyn-van Vliet FAC, van der Graaf Y, Bartelds AIM (1994) Prospective study of sentinel headache in aneurysmal subarachnoid haemorrhage. *The Lancet* **344**: 590–3.

Linn FHH, Rinkel GJE, Algra A, van Gijn J (1998) Headache characteristics in subarachnoid haemorrhage and benign thunderclap headache. *J Neurol Neurosurg Psychiatry* **65**: 791–3.

Morgenstern LB, Luna-Gonzales H, Huber JC, Jr, *et al.* (1998) Worst headache and subarachnoid hemorrhage: prospective, modern computed tomography and spinal fluid analysis. *Annals of Emergency Medicine* **32**: 297–304.

Newland C, Illis LS, Robinson PK, Batchelor BG, Waters WE (1978) A survey of headache in an English city. *Res Clin Stud Headache* **5**: 1–20.

Case 3 A woman with chest pain

Brenda was 40 when she consulted Dr Marks with a cough and right submammary pain. Two weeks previously she had recently returned from a month's holiday in Brazil where she had been treated for a chest infection with two courses of antibiotics. Dr Marks noted that Brenda felt slightly short of breath. She was taking the combined oral contraceptive (COCP), was a nonsmoker, and had a body mass index of 24.1. Her blood pressure was 159/95 and there were some crepitations at the right base. Dr Marks made a diagnosis of 'pleurisy' without recording any further detail about the pain.

What other information would you obtain?

Brenda told Dr Marks that she had had chest radiographs in Brazil that showed a lung infection. There was no observable calf or thigh swelling.

What would be your differential diagnosis and how would you discriminate between them?

A few days later Brenda became increasingly troubled by her chest pain and shortness of breath and went to A&E. She was admitted to hospital. Both the junior doctors who initially saw her suspected a pulmonary embolus. Brenda told them her pain had first occurred shortly after her flight to Brazil, and that her leg had swelled up at the same time. The diagnosis was confirmed by CT pulmonary angiogram, which showed widespread multiple pulmonary emboli.

Brenda sued Dr Marks for failing to consider the possibility of a pulmonary embolus.

Do you think her claim will succeed?

Expert opinion

Chest pain and complaints of breathlessness are both common in general practice. In this case the pain was unilateral and pleuritic in nature (sharp, well localized in time and position and worse on inspiration). It was associated with breathlessness. The differential diagnosis in this case included:

- pneumonia
- pulmonary infarction (a consequence of pulmonary embolus)
- lung abscess
- bronchiectasis
- malignancy, e.g. bronchogenic carcinoma
- pneumpthorax
- asbestos pleural disease, including mesothelioma.

The reason Dr Marks made the diagnosis of 'pleurisy' (presumably infective) was probably Brenda's own account of having been diagnosed with a chest infection on holiday. Possibly because of this, Dr Marks did not record a thorough history of the timing and onset of the symptoms some 6 weeks earlier. He does not appear to have enquired about associated features such as haemoptysis. He prematurely fixed on the diagnosis of 'pleurisy' and did not consider a wide differential diagnosis to explain what the underlying cause of Brenda's chest pain was.

Pulmonary emboli are relatively rare in general practice. The quoted incidence of pulmonary emboli is 25 per 100 000 per year. Thus a general practitioner with a list of 2000 will see one case every two years. According to Dalen and Master (2002):

It is well-recognized that the signs and symptoms of pulmonary embolism are nonspecific

Avoiding Errors in General Practice, First Edition. Kevin Barraclough, Jenny du Toit, Jeremy Budd, Joseph E. Raine, Kate Williams and Jonathan Bonser.
© 2013 John Wiley & Sons, Ltd. Published 2013 by John Wiley & Sons, Ltd.

and that, as a result, the clinical recognition of pulmonary embolism is notoriously inaccurate. The lack of sensitivity of the clinical diagnosis of pulmonary embolism is evident from post-mortem studies demonstrating that the majority of cases of pulmonary embolism detected post-mortem were not diagnosed (or treated) prior to death.

It is estimated in the USA that only 26% of pulmonary emboli are diagnosed and treated. 74% of cases are undiagnosed or diagnosed only after death (Dalen and Master, 2002).

In the Prospective Investigation of Pulmonary Embolism Diagnosis study (PIOPED) of the patients who survived long enough to have their pulmonary emboli diagnosed by pulmonary angiography (Stein & Henry, 1997):

- 65% presented with 'classical' symptoms of pulmonary infarction (death of lung tissue due to the clot). These probably represent the smallest volume emboli that fragment and impact in the distal bronchial tree (Ryu *et al.*, 1998).
- 22% presented with isolated breathlessness and no other features. Angiographic studies suggest that these are due to intermediate sized emboli that lodge in the pulmonary tree without producing infarction but significantly affect gas exchange and cause some degree of, possibly transitory, pulmonary hypertension (Ryu *et al.*, 1998).
- 8% presented with circulatory collapse. These are the large emboli that break off from the deep pelvic veins and impact at the principle trunks of the pulmonary artery. They present with the features described by Virchow: severe acute breathlessness, poorly localized chest pain and distress (probably from right ventricular distension and ischaemia), syncope or pre syncope, followed by recovery (if the patient survives) (Ryu *et al.*, 1998).
- 5% had no symptoms at all and were diagnosed on the basis of clinical suspicion after an abnormal chest X-ray (Ryu *et al.*, 1998).

Most clinicians (and all clinical prediction rules) rely significantly on the presence of risk factors to alert the doctor to the possibility of pulmonary embolism in clinically unobvious cases.

The British Thoracic Guideline for the management of suspected pulmonary embolism (June 2003) gives a list of risk factors and divides them into major risk factors (increasing the risk by a factor of 5 to 20) and minor risk factors (increasing risk by a factor of 2 to 4)

Case Table 3.1 Risk factors for venous thromboembolism.

Major risk factors (relative risk 5–20)	
Surgery[a]	• Major abdominal/pelvic surgery • Hip/knee replacement • Postoperative intensive care
Obstetrics	• Late pregnancy • Caesarian section • Puerperium
Lower limb problems	• Fracture • Varicose veins
Malignancy	• Abdominal/pelvic • Advanced/metastatic
Reduced mobility	• Hospitalization • Institutional care
Miscellaneous	• Previous VTE

Minor risk factors (relative risk 2–4)	
Cardiovascular	• Congenital heart disease • Congestive cardiac failure • Hypertension • Superficial venous thrombosis • Indwelling central vein catheter
Oestrogens	• Oral contraceptive • Hormone replacement therapy
Miscellaneous	• COPD • Neurological disability • Thrombotic disorders • Long-distance sedentary travel • Obesity • Other[b]

[a]Where appropriate prophlaxis is used, relative risk is much lower.
[b]Inflammatory bowel disease, nephrotic syndrome, chronic dialysis, myeloproliferative disorders, paroxysmal nocturnal haemoglobinuria, Behçet's disease.

(British Thoracic Society, 2003). This is reproduced as Case Table 3.1 .

A recent history of long-haul air travel is widely considered to increase the risk of venous thromboembolism. The evidence is effectively reviewed in the NHS Clinical knowledge summaries (NHS, 2011). In reality only a small proportion (about 1 in 4000–5000 flights) of air travellers have a deep vein thrombosis as a result. However, use of the combined oral contraceptive, obesity, Factor V Leiden mutation and extreme height increase this risk. The World Health Organization data estimated the odds ratio for the use of the COCP when flying to be 40. Therefore the prior probability of Brenda having a PE could have been as high as 1%.

The difficulty arises when patients do not present with the 'classical symptoms' of pulmonary embolism result from pulmonary infarction:

- pleuritic chest pain (sharp, well localized chest pain occurring on breathing in)
- cough
- haemoptysis
- tachycardia
- tachypnoea.

In this case Brenda does not seem to have had haemptoysis, although it may not have been recorded. However the persistence of symptoms of chest pain and shortness of breath over a six-week period was rather atypical for a previous diagnosis of chest infection. While pulmonary embolus is an uncommon diagnosis in general practice it should have been considered because of this combination of symptoms.

Thromboembolic disease is one of the top three medical causes of litigation against GPs. Cases tend to involve important disputes of fact about what history was given by the patient, or ought to have been elicited by a competent GP. It is also common for there to be an allegation that the GP simply failed to think of the possibility of thromboembolic disease. Both of these criticisms potentially apply in this case.

Should scoring systems be used to define risk? The Wells Rule (Wells *et al.*, 2000) is quite well known and may even be adopted for local care pathways between primary and secondary care. However it should be borne in mind that these scoring systems have been derived from populations presenting in secondary care in whom pulmonary embolus (or deep vein thrombosis as the case may be) have already been considered as a diagnosis. They have therefore not been validated for use in primary care. The AMUSE study has validated a Clinical Prediction Rule for use in primary care but relies heavily upon and requires a D Dimer result (Buller *et al.*, 2009).

 Legal comment

It is suggested by the legal expert that Dr Marks failed in his duty because he did not elicit an adequate history.

If he had elicited information that Brenda's pain came on shortly after her flight to Brazil and that her leg had swelled up at the same time, then he would have surely been alerted to the potential diagnosis of pulmonary embolism.

The number of potential diagnoses for chest pain and breathlessness make it incumbent on a GP to explore the patient's history carefully. It would therefore be difficult for a lawyer to obtain a contrary expert opinion.

We are not told what the outcome was for Brenda. Assuming successful treatment, she will have a claim for any pain or suffering before her problem was correctly diagnosed and treated. Since this was only a few days after the consultation, it would seem that this is a relatively small claim against Dr Marks, perhaps £2000–£3000.

 Key learning points

Specific to the case
- Always include pulmonary embolus in the differential diagnosis of pleuritic chest pain.
- In the absence of clear pointers to the diagnosis of pulmonary embolus, a key feature is the plausibility of the alternative diagnosis.
- If, as in this case, the diagnosis that was made was not plausible, there may be difficulty in defending the medical management.

General points
- It is good practice to always 'second guess' a presumed diagnosis.
- Is the presumed diagnosis the most likely?
- Is there another diagnosis that one 'cannot afford to miss'?

References and further reading

British Thoracic Society Standards of Care Committee Pulmonary Embolism Guideline Development Group (2003) British Thoracic Society guidelines for the management of suspected acute pulmonary embolism. *Thorax* **58**: 470–83.

Buller HR, Cate-Hoek AJ, Hoes AW, *et al.* (2009) Safely ruling out deep venous thrombosis in primary care *Annals of Internal Medicine* **150**: 229–35.

Dalen M, Master M (2002) Pulmonary embolism: What have we learnt since Virchow? Natural history, pathophysiology and diagnosis. *Chest* **122**: 1440–56.

Meyer G, Roy P-M, Gilberg S, Perrier A (2010) Easily missed? Pulmonary embolism. *BMJ* **340**: c1421.

NHS (2011) Clinical knowledge summaries http://www.cks.nhs.uk/dvt_prevention_for_travellers/evidence/supporting_evidence/risk_of_travel_related_dvt#-390015

Ryu J, Jay H, Olson EJ, Pellikka PA (1998) Clinical recognition of pulmonary embolism: problem of unrecognized and asymptomatic cases. *Mayo Clinic Proceedings* **73**: 873–9.

Stein PD, Henry J (1997) Clinical characteristics of patients with acute pulmonary embolism stratified according to their presenting symptoms. *Chest* **112**: 974–80.

Wells PS, Anderson DR, Rodger M, Ginsberg JS, Kearon C, Gent M, *et al.* (2000) Derivation of a simple clinical model to categorize patients probability of pulmonary embolism: increasing the models utility with the SimpliRED D-dimer. *Thromb Haemost* **83**: 416–20.

Case 4 A dizzy man

Bernard was 60 years old when he was visited by an Out of Hours general practitioner, Dr Carter, on a weekend evening. He stated that he woke that day, turned over in bed and felt that the room was spinning. He had vomited twice in the bed. During the morning he felt unsteady on his feet and had become very anxious because he lived on his own and was unsure how he would cope. He had felt nonspecifically unwell for a couple of days with a sore throat and malaise. He had made himself some hot lemon with whisky that evening but had been unable to drink it. He had had a coronary angioplasty and stent two years earlier and was on a statin, aspirin and a beta blocker.

What would you do now?

Dr Carter established that the vertigo was intermittently so severe that Bernard had difficulty standing. He had difficulty walking but managed if he kept his head still. He felt comfortable once he was sitting still or lying down. On direct questioning he had a slight headache, was not aware of any weakness, had a sore throat and a hoarse voice.

What would be your differential diagnosis and how would you discriminate between them?

Dr Carter noted that the man looked well but anxious, had a temperature of 37.4 °C, pulse 64/min regular and a BP 174/92 mmHg. Dr Carter suggested doing a Hallpike test but Bernard was anxious about provoking the vertigo. Dr Carter recorded that Bernard probably had a viral labyrinthitis and pharyngitis and prescribed stemetil and paracetamol.

Bernard's son visited him the next day and found his father was unwell with a high fever and a severe cough. He took him to the local ED department where a chest X-ray demonstrated a pneumonia. He was admitted onto a general medical ward. The following day one of the nurses noted that Bernard was choking when drinking fluids. Further assessment by the medical registrar demonstrated that the man had a hoarse voice, a weak cough and that palatal movements were asymmetric on saying 'aah' (the uvula moving to the left). Bernard regurgitated water on drinking. Light touch was subjectively different on the right cheek to the left, there was a right Horner's syndrome, sustained nystagmus and he could not walk unaided. A cranial MRI scan demonstrated patchy infarction of the right lateral medulla and inferior cerebellum. The diagnosis was made of an aspiration pneumonia secondary to a brainstem stroke. Bernard was unwell and dehydrated and his neurological deficit extended. A further MRI showed more extensive dorsolateral medullary infarction. Bernard made only a partial recovery.

Bernard sued Dr Carter for failing to consider the possibility of a stroke and for omitting to check for dysphagia, and sued the hospital for initially missing the stroke and treating him for pneumonia.

Do you think his claim will succeed?

Expert opinion

Vertigo is a difficult presentation for a general practitioner and requires careful assessment. It is relatively common. A full time general practitioner can expect to see 10–20 cases of acute vertigo per year (McCormick et al., 1995). The vast majority will be due to malfunctions of the labyrinth – vertigo caused by a peripheral lesion. Roughly 40% will be due to benign paroxysmal positional vertigo (BPPV), 40% will be due to acute vestibular neuritis and a significant proportion of the rest may have vestibular migraine (Barraclough &

Avoiding Errors in General Practice, First Edition. Kevin Barraclough, Jenny du Toit, Jeremy Budd, Joseph E. Raine, Kate Williams and Jonathan Bonser.
© 2013 John Wiley & Sons, Ltd. Published 2013 by John Wiley & Sons, Ltd.

Bronstein, 2009). However, a critical aspect of the general practitioner's assessment must be to distinguish the tiny number of cases of vertigo due to brainstem lesions (mostly brainstem strokes) from the large number of peripheral causes of vertigo.

In this case there were a number of features that should have alerted Dr Carter to consider the possibility of a central (brain stem) cause rather than a peripheral cause. At 60 Bernard was in the age range where cerebrovascular events are not uncommon. It was a concern that he had difficulty walking and drinking and that his voice was hoarse. The latter were suggestive of dysphagia and dysphonia.

Dr Carter should have established a few additional features. It was not clear from the history if the vertigo was positional or sustained. He should have seen if the man could drink a glass of water. If he could drink then significant dysphagia was unlikely. He should have seen him walk and checked that there was no facial, hand or arm weakness. All these are quite easy tests and if normal, make a brainstem stroke unlikely. If the tests were abnormal the man should have been referred immediately into hospital with a possible stroke (NICE, July 2008, Clinical guidelines on stroke).

Because structures in the brainstem are closely packed together, vertigo in the absence of any other cranial nerve features (such as diplopia, facial weakness, facial numbness, dysphagia, dysphonia) or long tract symptoms (such as weakness or numbness of the limbs) is unlikely to be due to a central cause. Fewer than 1% of 407 patients with posterior circulation strokes in the New England Medical Centre Posterior Circulation Registry (NEMC-PCR) presented with a single isolated symptom (Caplan *et al.*, 2004). Another study of 1666 patients aged over 44 presenting to a US emergency department with 'dizziness' found 53 (3.6%) were due to a stroke or a TIA. In patients with 'dizziness' without other symptoms or signs only 0.7% had had a stroke or TIA (Kerber *et al.*, 2006).

Dr Carter attempted to make a positive diagnosis but was negligent in not checking that there were no other neurological signs – particularly dysphagia, dysphonia, palatal weakness, facial weakness or numbness or ataxia.

 ## Legal comment

The expert says it was negligent of Dr Carter not to have checked Bernard for neurological signs. If he had done so, he would have probably found abnormalities which would have led him to admit Bernard to hospital.

As it was, in the hours before his son came to visit, it seems that Bernard developed an aspiration pneumonia because of his dysphagia. That pneumonia may have worsened the neurological deficit which will now affect Bernard for the rest of his life. He has sued both the GP and the hospital.

As well as looking at breach of duty the lawyers for each will take expert opinions on the cause of the additional neurological deficit. Maybe after all, despite any failings by either party, that deficit is entirely unrelated. It may have been simply a continuation of the brain stem infarction. In that case, Bernard's claim will fail.

But if Bernard's worse outcome is probably the result of the aspiration pneumonia, then Dr Carter's MDO will have to pay Bernard compensation to reflect his additional disabilities.

The MDO may seek a contribution from the hospital. If there is expert medical evidence to suggest that it too was negligent then there is likely to be negotiation between the lawyers for those two defendants.

Bernard's compensation will be assessed according to a comparison between the likely outcome if he had been properly managed, and the actual outcome. The costs of any additional care now required because of the additional deficit will be calculated by reference to Bernard's life expectancy.

 ## Key learning points

Specific to the case
• In cases of acute vertigo it is essential to consider the possibility of a brainstem stroke.
• Check the onset and duration of the vertigo and whether it is positional or not. Check that there is no headache or hearing loss.
• On examination check eye movements and nystagmus (should be horizontal only and ideally whether the pupils are equal. Check there is no facial weakness, dyaphagia or dysphonia. Check for gait or limb ataxia and look in the ears for a cholesteatoma.

General points
• It is always necessary to be wary of subtle details that 'do not fit'.

References and further reading

Barraclough K, Bronstein A (2009) Diagnosis in general practice: vertigo, *BMJ* **339**: 749–52.

Caplan L, Chung C-S, Wityk R, *et al.* (2004) New England Medical Center Posterior Circulation Registry. *Annals of Neurology* **56**: 389–98.

Kerber KA, Brown DL, Lisabeth LD, Smith MA, Morgenstern LB (2006) Stroke among patients with dizziness, vertigo, and imbalance in the emergency department: a population-based study. *Stroke* **37**: 2484–7.

McCormick A, Fleming D, Charlton J (1995) *Morbidity Statistics from General Practice: Fourth National Study, 1991–1992.* London, Office of Population Censuses and Surveys.

NICE (2008) Diagnosis and initial management of acute stroke and transient ischaemic attack (TIA), Clinical guidelines CG68, July 2008.

Case 5 Rectal bleeding in a pregnant woman

Sadie, a 38-year-old woman in her third pregnancy, attended the practice antenatal clinic at 32 weeks mentioned to her midwife that she had occasional bleeding from her back passage. She had had problems with 'piles' since her second pregnancy two years earlier. The midwife thought that she probably had piles again but suggested that she saw her GP.

If you had been her GP what would you have done?

Two weeks later Sadie saw Dr Arnold but was more concerned about severe heartburn. She mentioned that she was having trouble with her piles. The Dr Arnold prescribed Anusol and an antacid.

Sadie consulted a different GP in the practice, Dr Durrant, a month later because she was worried that the bleeding from her back passage was happening more frequently. The blood was on the paper and in the pan. She experienced discomfort when opening her bowels. She had been constipated for a few weeks. She had the occasional abdominal pain that she attributed to everything stretching as the pregnancy progressed. Dr Durrant reassured her that there was nothing serious going on. He advised her to increase her fluid intake and gave her a prescription for some lactulose and proctosedyl suppositories.

Sadie had a normal vaginal delivery at term. She and the baby were seen for their postnatal check at eight weeks. She said that everything was fine and she had no particular problems.

Would you have done anything differently?

Nine months later Sadie sought help from Dr Bradley for continuing problems with her piles. She had had intermittent bright red blood on opening her bowels since giving birth although she had not mentioned it at her postnatal visit. She no longer had any anal symptoms. For the past month she had been opening her bowels more frequently. She had not had any diarrhoea. There was no family history of colorectal cancer. She was not anaemic. Abdominal examination was unremarkable. A rectal examination was normal. Dr Bradley performed routine blood tests including a viscosity. These were all normal. When on review two weeks later the symptoms were unchanged Dr Bradley referred Sadie under the 'Two week rule'. At colonoscopy there was a mid sigmoid colonic carcinoma.

Unfortunately histology following a left hemicolectomy showed local invasion and lymph node involvement. Sadie sued her GPs for delay in the diagnosis of her cancer and subsequent poor prognosis.

Expert opinion

Was the management of this patient reasonable or should she have been investigated sooner?

Studies have shown that rectal bleeding is common in the general population (Crosland & Jones, 1995). A questionnaire study of 6000 adult patients found that 26% of women under the age of 40 had experienced rectal bleeding in the previous 12 months (Thompson et al., 2000). Most patients do not present to doctors with their symptoms. This phenomenon, of the high frequency of symptoms in the community that are never reported to doctors, is often referred to as the 'Symptom Iceberg' (Hanny, 1979). One of the consequences of this 'Symptom Iceberg' is that patients who present to their doctor specifically with rectal bleeding are likely to have a much higher risk of having colorectal cancer (even though the risk may still be very low) than patients who do not volunteer the symptom but respond in the affirmative to a question (on a questionnaire or from a doctor) about whether or not they have experienced rectal bleeding.

Avoiding Errors in General Practice, First Edition. Kevin Barraclough, Jenny du Toit, Jeremy Budd, Joseph E. Raine, Kate Williams and Jonathan Bonser.
© 2013 John Wiley & Sons, Ltd. Published 2013 by John Wiley & Sons, Ltd.

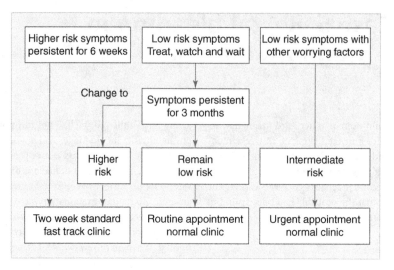

Case Figure 5.1 Algorithms for referral of patients with lower gastrointestinal symptoms.

A 2007 study by Roger Jones looked at a computerized database of 750 000 patients in primary care and found that 0.2% of women aged less than 45 with rectal bleeding had colorectal cancer (CRC) (Jones *et al.*, 2007). Lewis *et al* (2002) estimated that the prevalence of undiagnosed CRC in a 35 year old presenting with rectal bleeding is 1 in 11 574.

It could be argued that it would have been prudent to perform a proctoscopy to confirm the presence of piles. However, in 1992 a survey showed that only 70% of general practices possessed proctoscopes and, in those practices that did, only three-quarters of the doctors used them (Rubin, 1995). It is unlikely that a GP would perform a proctoscopy late in the third trimester of pregnancy. Had the GP reviewed the woman's recent past history and enquired about her rectal bleeding at the postnatal check, they might have done a proctoscopy. In this case, finding piles, which can co-exist with colorectal carcinoma, would have given false reassurance. However it would have enabled the GP to provide further treatment and arrange appropriate follow up and safety netting.

Managing a patient with rectal bleeding, who falls within 'Two Week Rule' guidance, is straightforward. This case illustrates the difficulty posed by low risk patients. Rectal bleeding with anal symptoms (such as discomfort) is considered 'Low Risk' at any age. The April 2002 Health Referral Guidelines for Bowel Cancer state (p. 36): 'Rectal bleeding as a single symptom is of little diagnostic value. Its value is increased when it occurs

in association with a change in bowel habit and when it occurs without anal symptoms.' Thompson *et al.* (2003) has outlined a 'Treat, watch and wait' policy for patients with low risk symptoms (rectal bleeding with an anal cause and no change in bowel habit to loose frequent stools). This management plan is illustrated in Case Figure 5.1 from the August 2003 article by Thompson.

In this case the difficulty is to decide where the 3-month review period starts. The patient should have either been reviewed or asked to make an appointment to a doctor again if her symptoms did not improve between one and three months after her postnatal visit. If her rectal bleeding persisted and she had not developed any high risk symptoms she should have been referred for non-urgent investigations.

 Legal comment

In order to succeed in her claim, Sadie will have to show that there has been a breach of duty by one or more of the GPs who saw her over the period in question.

To do that, she must obtain an expert opinion (by a GP) which highlights a failing. The expert will have to say that there is no responsible body of medical opinion specialized in general practice which would have acted in the way the GP did. In this scenario, it seems unlikely that Sadie will be able to get such an opinion.

Before the birth, it seems most GPs would not have done a proctoscopy. At the postnatal check, there was no complaint of rectal bleeding to prompt such an examination, and anyway it seems that a substantial body of GPs would not have done a proctoscopy anyway. The best that can be said is that if there had been a complaint of rectal bleeding, Sadie may have been encouraged to come back to the GP sooner than she did. In turn, that may have led to a chain of events whereby the cancer was detected sooner, and the prognosis was better.

But, as it is, it seems unlikely that Sadie will be able to get a sufficiently supportive medical report to justify issuing proceedings.

 Key learning points

Specific to the case
- Colorectal cancer in patients under the age of 45 years is extremely rare.
- It is important to safety net and have some sort of follow up arrangement for patients with low-risk symptoms for colorectal cancer.

General points
- If the likelihood of a disease is low it may be reasonable that the diagnosis is delayed.

References and further reading

Crosland A, Jones R (1995) Rectal bleeding: prevalence and consultation behaviour. *BMJ* **311**: 486–8.

Hanny DR (1979) *The Symptoms Iceberg: A Study Of Community Health*. London: Routledge & Kegan Paul.

Jones R, Latinovic R, Charlton J, Gulliford MC (2007) Alarm symptoms in early diagnosis of cancer in primary care: cohort study using General Practice Research Database. *BMJ* **334**: 1040.

Lewis JD, Brown A, Locallo AR, Schwartz J (2002) Initial evaluation of rectal bleeding in young persons: a cost-effectiveness analysis. *Annals of Internal Medicine* **136**(2): 99–110.

Rubin GP (1995) Endoscopy facilities in general practice. *BMJ* **304**: 1542–3.

Thompson JA, Pond CL, Ellis BG, Beach A, Thompson MR (2000) Rectal bleeding in general and hospital practice; 'the tip of the iceberg'. *Colorectal Disease* **2**: 288–93.

Thompson MR, Heath I, Ellis BG, Swarbrick ET, Faulds Wood L, Atkin WS (2003) Identifying and managing patients at low risk of bowel cancer in general practice. *BMJ* **327**: 263–5.

Case 6 A pulled calf muscle

Cheryl, aged 32, consulted Dr David in the Out of Hours service on a Saturday morning with a two-day history of a painful left calf. She was concerned as to whether it could be a DVT because she was on the oral contraceptive pill and was due to fly to Tenerife that afternoon for a holiday. She had played basket ball on the previous Tuesday evening (to which she was unaccustomed) but had not noted any injury, though she had felt generally stiff the next day.

What are the clinical features that you would consider discriminatory when assessing a possible DVT?

Dr David established that Cheryl had no past history of DVT. An aunt had had a 'blood clot' at some stage. Cheryl was a light smoker. On examination the left calf was tender to deep palpation, particularly in one spot. Dr David thought the calf might be a little swollen. There was moderate pitting oedema of the left ankle and a scrap of pitting oedema at the right ankle. Cheryl explained that she did get 'water retention' on the pill.

What would you do now?

Dr David stated that he did not think that Cheryl had a DVT but that he could not exclude it. He advised that he could send Cheryl to the hospital for tests but she was anxious not to miss her holiday. They agreed that if the calf became more painful or more swollen Cheryl would seek medical help in Tenerife.

After a few days on holiday her left leg was significantly more swollen and she attended the hospital. There was a 4 cm difference in calf circumference, her D Dimer was very raised and ultrasound demonstrated evidence of extensive thrombus in the left distal superficial and popliteal veins. Despite anticoagulation Cheryl has been told that she is at risk of developing the post phlebitic syndrome. She has brought an action against Dr David alleging that he failed to appropriately manage her condition on the Saturday and send her to hospital.

Do you think her claim will succeed?

 Expert opinion

Delayed or missed diagnoses of DVTs and pulmonary emboli are common causes of actions against general practitioners. The difficulty is that lower leg swelling and pain are both relatively common findings in primary care and are usually not due to DVT.

DVT is frequently suspected in young women on the oral contraceptive pill but clearly, many women are on the pill and few get DVTs. The relative risk of having a DVT on the oral contraceptive pill is about three times that of the background population. This compares with a figure of over 20 in patients after major surgery (Chunilal et al., 2003). However, the absolute risk of DVT is low, at about 1 per 1000 per year (doubling after the age of 70). In a 32-year-old woman the incidence remains very low, whether she is taking the oral contraceptive pill or not.

In view of the fact that the clinical suspicion and diagnosis of DVT is difficult there have been various clinical prediction rules that have developed to try and increase the accuracy of diagnosis. The most widely used in hospital is probably the 'Well's Score' (Wells et al., 2006). This is reproduced in Case Table 6.1.

There is necessarily an aspect of subjective clinical judgment because of the question about whether another diagnosis is more likely. However, a particular difficulty is that prospective trials have given quite different predictive values for patients with different scores. In the original study 16% of the study population had DVT and 75% of those with a score of 3 or above had DVT and only 3% of those with a score of zero or less. A meta analysis gave values of 53% (score 3 or more)

Avoiding Errors in General Practice, First Edition. Kevin Barraclough, Jenny du Toit, Jeremy Budd, Joseph E. Raine, Kate Williams and Jonathan Bonser.
© 2013 John Wiley & Sons, Ltd. Published 2013 by John Wiley & Sons, Ltd.

Case Table 6.1 Simplified clinical model for assessment of deep vein thrombosis.*

Clinical Variable	Score
Active cancer (treatment ongoing or within previous 6 months or palliative)	1
Paralysis, paresis, or recent plaster Immobilization of the lower extremIties	1
Recently bedridden for 3 days or more, or major surgery within the previous 12 weeks requiring general or regional anesthesia	1
Localized tenderness along the distribution of the deep venous system	1
Entire leg swelling	1
Calf swelling at least 3 cm larger than that on the asymptomatic leg (measured 10 cm below the tibial tuberosity)†	1
Pitting edema confined to the symptomatic leg	1
Collateral superficial veins (nonvaricose)	1
Previously documented DVT	1
Alternative diagnosis at least as likely as DVT	−2

Abbreviation: DVT, deep vein thrombosis.
*Scoring method indicates high probability if score is 3 or more; moderate if score is 1 or 2; and low if score is 0 or less,
†In patients with symptoms in both legs, the more symptomatic leg was used.

and 5% (zero or less). A Dutch primary care study with an overall probability of DVT of 29% gave rather disappointing figures of 37.5% (3 or more) and still 12% for a score of zero or less. Thus the role of the Wells Score in primary care remains rather uncertain.

In practice, a general practitioner should probably gather the information that is shown to be discriminatory in the Wells Score, request a D Dimer test only if the Wells Score is zero or less (when negative D Dimer should rule the diagnosis out with a probability of DVT of only 0.3%) and otherwise refer for imaging and assessment if the Wells score is 1 or more or there is clinical suspicion and a D Dimer is unavailable.

This case illustrates several of the problems that occur quite frequently in medico-legal cases.

One issue is the question of informed consent. Dr David recorded that he 'offered' to send Cheryl to hospital but that she decided against it. Her decision only absolves Cheryl of liability if she was fully informed by Dr David of the consequences of her decision. To give consent in law the patient must have been told all the risks that a reasonable person would consider might influence their decision. In practice it is rare to see documented evidence of such 'informed dissent'.

In this case it would have been necessary to tell Cheryl that there was some degree of risk that she may have a DVT and that if it was undiagnosed it could lead to death from pulmonary embolism or disability from pulmonary embolism or DVT. Cheryl argued that she would not have taken the decision to fly if she had been so informed.

The second issue is the question of measurement and documentation. Dr David recorded that the calf was 'a little swollen'. Clearly this is a less specific bit of information than a recorded circumference taken 10 cm below the tibial tuberosity. Furthermore, since there is evidence that a difference in circumference of more than 3 cm is significant and of less is not, a general practitioner is arguably obliged to make use of that specific bit of information in a clinical situation in which diagnosis is difficult. It would be difficult to argue that Dr David's assessment was thorough when it would have been easy to carry out the measurement, helpfully discriminatory and it is widespread practice.

A further difficulty was that history to suggest any alternative cause (a gastrocnemius strain or tear) was poor. It was not plausible that Cheryl's symptoms starting two days later were due to an unnoticed calf strain when playing basket ball.

Cheryl's Wells Score would probably have been 3 if Dr David had measured her calf and her probability of having a DVT was probably 30% to 60%, but certainly not insignificant.

In this case these factors would make it not possible to defend an allegation of breach of duty.

 Legal comment

Cheryl's lawyers will approach a GP for an expert report on whether Dr David was in breach of his duty to her. They will provide their expert with a written statement by Cheryl and with Dr David's records of the consultation. The expert's report will be based on this evidence.

In her witness statement, Cheryl will describe the consultation. She will recall the advice Dr David gave her on whether to go to Tenerife that afternoon or go to hospital for some tests. It seems that Dr David did not give her adequate advice about the risk she was taking by not going for tests, and that if he had, she would have stayed for the tests. Unless he has adequately recorded his advice about the risks she ran, Dr David will be at a significant disadvantage in the proceedings.

Thus the success of Cheryl's litigation will turn on the facts, and whether the Judge believes her or Dr David.

In those circumstances, Dr David's MDO is likely to wish to settle the case rather than take the risk of going to trial. After all, this may not be a very expensive case to settle – Cheryl is to be compensated for the pain and suffering which she would not otherwise have had, and that was only for a few days until she got treatment. Cheryl may be entitled to compensation if she can show that she is more likely than not to develop post-phlebitic syndrome and that this was due to Dr David's failure to properly advise.

References and further reading

Chunilal SD, Eikelboom JW, Attia J, Miniati M, Panju AA, Simel DL *et al.* (2003) Does this patient have pulmonary embolism? *JAMA* **290**: 2849–58.

Wells PS, Owen C, Doucette S, Fergusson D, Tran H (2006) Does this patient have deep vein thrombosis? *JAMA* **295**: 199–207.

 Key learning points

Specific to the case

• When assessing a possible DVT the most highly discriminating factors are those listed in the Wells Score. It is important to make sure that these bits of information are elicited and recorded.

• Only request a D Dimer test (if available) if the Wells Score is zero or less. Only then will a negative result effectively exclude the probability of DVT. If the Wells Score is 1 or more refer for imaging in hospital.

• If there is a significant possibility of DVT and a D Dimer is not available then refer to hospital.

General points

• When a patient declines to follow advice, or makes a decision against treatment or referral, it is important to make sure (and document) that the patient is fully informed about the consequences of such a decision.

Case 7 A woman with hemiplegic migraine

A 40-year-old woman, Jane, presented to a general practitioner, Dr Allen, on a Monday morning. On the previous Saturday she had been shopping with her sister when she began to feel unwell. She had had pain in her neck and the back of her head, nausea and felt clammy. Her sister had found her a seat in the shopping mall. Her sister wondered if Jane was having a panic attack, as this had happened before. Her lips and tongue became tingly and her left arm became numb. A passer-by had been called and helped Jane back to the car. Her sister drove her home and Jane spent the day in bed with a severe headache. The following day (Sunday) Jane was much better, though she still had severe headache and neck ache. By Monday she was feeling considerably better. Dr Allen noted that Jane had a history of anxiety and depression, had been taking citalopram but had recently stopped and had been prescribed sumatriptan in the past.

What would you do now?

Dr Allen checked Jane's pulse, blood pressure, fundoscopy, walking and the power in her arms, all of which were normal. Dr Allen wondered about a diagnosis of hemiplegic migraine, possibly related to stopping the citalopram, arranged some blood tests, prescribed a tryptan in wafer form plus some tramadol and arranged review in a week. In a week Jane was better.

What would be your differential diagnosis and how would you discriminate between them?

Two months later Jane returned to see Dr Bendick, who was an ST3 general practitioner registrar in the practice. Dr Allen was his trainer. Jane had had two episodes in the interim where she had had headache and numbness affecting her right arm and leg. These had been less severe than the first episode but had scarred her as she had wondered if she was having a stroke. The numbness had lasted a day or so and headache had lasted several days, though it was only severe for a day or so. Examination was normal.

Dr Bendick decided to ask Dr Allen. Dr Allen felt that the diagnosis was hemiplegic migraine. They were initially going to prescribe propanolol but Jane pointed out that she had been told not to take propanolol (which she had been prescribed for panic attacks in the past), because she had asthma. Dr Bendrick found asthma medication in the past drugs. Dr Allen suggested pizotifen instead. Two weeks later Dr Bendick reviewed Jane. She had had no further episodes since taking the pizotifen. Dr Bendick advised continuing the pizotifen for 3 months.

Three weeks later Jane collapsed while watching her daughter's school play. She was admitted to hospital by emergency ambulance and a head CT scan showed a large right intracerebral haemorrhage thought to be due to an arteriovenous malformation. Jane died two days later on ITU.

Jane's husband brought a claim against Dr Bendick and Dr Allen. It was alleged that the diagnosis of hemiplegic migraine was unsafe, that the history recorded was insufficiently detailed and did not accord with Jane's sister's account, that Jane was taking the combined oral contraceptive pill and that this should have been stopped, and that Jane should have been referred into hospital with the first and subsequent episodes.

Do you think his claim will succeed?

 ## Expert opinion

The diagnosis of hemiplegic migraine was not implausible but unfortunately it was clearly unsafe (Black, 2006; NICE, 2008). There were also other oversights in Jane's management which, while they did not directly cause her harm, would be likely to be considered by the Court to be indicative of substandard practice.

Avoiding Errors in General Practice, First Edition. Kevin Barraclough, Jenny du Toit, Jeremy Budd, Joseph E. Raine, Kate Williams and Jonathan Bonser.
© 2013 John Wiley & Sons, Ltd. Published 2013 by John Wiley & Sons, Ltd.

Dr Allen recorded a history of transient neurological dysfunction associated with headache. However, there was little recorded detail about duration of symptoms and no detail about the onset of the headache. With any transient neurological symptom the detailed history is all important in making the diagnosis and needs to be recorded in significant detail.

It would have been good practice to attempt to get a telephone history from Jane's sister. This would have revealed that the onset of the headache was sudden, that Jane had had difficulty holding a water bottle in her left hand and had had difficulty walking to the car. There had been a suspicion of left-sided facial weakness and the weakness lasted several hours.

There was evidence in Dr Allen's witness statement that she was reassured by the fact that examination was normal and by the fact that Jane had a past history of classical migraine. However, it is clear that transient neurological symptoms can still be due to serious underlying disease and that Jane's history of classical migraine still only marginally increased the likelihood that the diagnosis was hemiplegic migraine but that, critically, it did not make the presumptive diagnosis a safe one. Hemiplegic migraine is one of those diagnoses that, although it figures prominently in medical teaching and textbooks, is rare.

Dr Allen was inappropriately reassured and she did not consider the necessary differential diagnoses.

If Dr Allen had looked up migraine using medical web resources she would have read that it may sometimes be safe to ascribe fully reversible hemisensory symptoms that resolve in 5–60 minutes to migraine, if the time course of the aura and headache is typical and there is a suggestive past history, but it is never safe to ascribe motor symptoms to migraine without specialist investigation to exclude other causes such as TIAs, subarachnoid haemorrhages or vasoactive tumours.

Dr Allen appears to have 'prematurely anchored' on the hypothesis of hemiplegic migraine and failed to consider the other possibilities.

As is often the case when a diagnosis has been made in an unsafe manner, the problem was compounded because subsequent clinicians assume it is correct. In this case Dr Bendick assumed that the diagnosis was correct. Dr Bendick, as a trainee, would be assessed by the standard of a reasonably competent fully qualified colleague.

It is relatively common that, even in training practices, careful scrutiny reveals that there are significant failings in the summarized past medical history. In this case it should have been recorded that Jane had a past history of asthma. This had already nearly resulted in

significant error when Jane had been prescribed beta blockers for anxiety but had still not been recorded on the summary. Neither Dr Allen nor Dr Bendick had established that Jane was taking the combined pill, which is contraindicated with focal migraine. The Claimant experts were critical of these failings even though they led to no harm.

 Legal comment

It seems that Jane's family will be able to establish that Dr Allen was negligent in not referring her for specialist investigation after the first consultation. She also should have stopped the oral contraceptive pill. Dr Allen's initial negligence was continued by Dr Bendrick at subsequent consultations. He had two opportunities to refer Jane, but did not take them. The fact that he is only a trainee does not mean he is judged by a lower standard. He is judged by the standard of the ordinary competent GP (see Expert comment above).

The two doctors' MDOs will wish to investigate what the outcome would probably have been if Jane had been referred at the first consultation. In investigating causation, their expert will be asked to consider the following questions: when would she have been investigated, and what would the investigations have shown?; what treatment would have been given?; would death have probably been avoided?

If the answer to this last question is yes, then Jane's husband and children will have a good claim. They will be entitled to bereavement damages of £11 800 and a sum representing the unnecessary pain and suffering she experienced before she died. Her children will have a claim for the loss of their mother's love, care and support during their childhood. Her husband will have a claim to cover the loss of the care Jane provided to him. The family will also be entitled to compensation representing her financial contribution to the household.

The value of this claim will depend on Jane's earning power and other features of her family life, but it will most likely be worth in excess of £100 000 and could be significantly more.

 Key learning points

Specific to the case
• It is unsafe to make a diagnosis of hemiplegic migraine without specialist assessment to exclude other causes of transient weakness.
• With any history of transient neurological symptoms it is always important to elicit and

record as much detail as possible about the event. Examination is usually unhelpful. If there is any possibility of doing so always attempt to speak to a witness directly.
• With any woman with a presumed diagnosis of focal migraine always ask about the pill, which may have been prescribed elsewhere.

General points
• When postulating a rare diagnosis it is always wise to check web resources on the web.
• Be very careful about accepting uncritically a diagnosis made earlier by a colleague (particularly if made in hospital by someone whose seniority is unknown).
• Significant diagnoses are often missed from medical summaries and can easily lead to error.

References and further reading

Black D (2006) Sporadic and familial hemiplegic migraine: diagnosis and treatment. *Semin Neurol* **26**: 208–16.

NICE (2008) Diagnosis and initial management of acute stroke and transient ischaemic attack (TIA), Clinical guidelines CG68, July 2008.

Online resources

British Association for the Study of Headaches and the International Headache Society: http://www.bash.org.uk/ and http://www.i-h-s.org/ – very good guidance on the assessment of headaches.

Case 8 Irritable bowel syndrome after sickness in Goa

Alison, a 51-year-old English teacher, consulted Dr Chowdury following a holiday in Goa. Towards the end of her holiday she had colicky lower abdominal pain and on her return to the UK she had developed diarrhoea. Dr Chowdury arranged for stool cultures and reviewed her by phone one week later. The diarrhoea had not settled and Alison had noticed blood in the stool. The stool cultures were negative. Dr Chowdury referred Alison to the gastroenterologists to exclude inflammatory bowel disease. However the patient did not attend the appointment, presumably because her symptoms settled.

Alison consulted Dr Browne six months later. She was complaining of diarrhoea four or five times a day for the previous two weeks. She had intermittent lower abdominal pain but no blood or mucus in the stool. She had not lost any weight. Dr Browne noted that Alison had had an episode of diarrhoea the previous year and although referred had not been investigated. The diarrhoea seemed to be associated with stress at work. He also recorded that there was no family history of inflammatory bowel disease or colorectal cancer. He did not examine Alison because she looked well.

What would be your differential diagnosis?

Dr Browne organized blood tests, gave Alison a prescription for loperamide and arranged to review her in two weeks.

A computer entry one week later recorded normal FBC, U&E, LFT and glucose. The viscosity was 1.91 and the CRP 83. The result was actioned as 'review as planned'.

Two days after the computer entry Alison attended a Walk in Centre because she felt worse. She had lost weight. The frequency of her diarrhoea had increased to 10 times a day and she had noticed blood in the stool. It was not clear whether she was assessed by a triage nurse or saw a doctor. An initial triage note recorded

that Alison looked 'pale and unwell'. Despite this a later consultation note recorded that she was 'systemically well', possibly because her temperature, pulse and blood pressure were normal. An abdominal examination was not performed. She was advised to see her own GP because of her persistent symptoms.

Alison returned to the practice for review three days later. She was seen by Dr White who noted a history of diarrhoea for two weeks with 'blood in the motions'. On examination: PR 84; BP 128/80; soft abdomen but left iliac fossa tenderness. Dr White did not record that she had seen the raised viscosity or CRP. The diagnosis was '? colitis'. Stool cultures were arranged and Alison was prescribed ciprofloxacin and advised to continue loperamide. A review appointment was made for three weeks.

What would you have done differently?

Two days later Alison was admitted to hospital by the Out of Hours service. On admission she was extremely unwell and a diagnosis of severe ulcerative colitis with a toxic megacolon was made. Alison had a total colectomy with necrotic bowel. Her postoperative recovery was complicated by septicaemia. She was discharged six weeks later.

Alison sued the three general practitioners and the practice. She argued that she had not been properly assessed, that a differential diagnosis of inflammatory bowel disease should have been considered and that the practice had neglected to deal competently with her abnormal blood results.

Expert opinion

Acute diarrhoea is an extremely common presentation in general practice. The HPA defines acute diarrhoea as three or more episodes of loose stool a day for less than 14 days (HPA, 2010).

Avoiding Errors in General Practice, First Edition. Kevin Barraclough, Jenny du Toit, Jeremy Budd, Joseph E. Raine, Kate Williams and Jonathan Bonser.

20% of the UK population experience gastroenteritis in any one year; 1 in 6 of those affected consults their GP (Wheeler et al., 1999). A study performed in the USA found gastroenteritis to be even more common, estimating 1.4 episodes of infective gastroenteritis per person per year (Herikstad et al., 2002).

The clinical features of infective gastroenteritis are abdominal pain, diarrhoea and vomiting. 76% of patients with infective diarrhoea no longer have symptoms after three weeks (Cumberland, 2003). The 1996 UK guideline on the management of infective gastroenteritis states: 'Most episodes of infective gastroenteritis last for less than 14 days. The risk of an underlying non-infective diagnosis and the need for further investigation both increase if symptoms are prolonged' (Farthing et al., 1996).

A competent general practitioner should take a careful history to elicit the duration and severity of the symptoms and the presence or absence of abdominal pain, nausea and vomiting, blood in the stool and weight loss. The examination should include an assessment of hydration, temperature, pulse, BP and abdominal palpation. It is generally only necessary to perform a rectal examination if there is rectal bleeding.

The vast majority of cases of infective gastroenteritis in adults require no investigation and no specific treatment other than advice about rehydration.

A review paper in 2009 in the *BMJ* on the management of acute diarrhoea (defined as diarrhoea lasting less than four weeks) makes the point that acute diarrhoea has a low predictive value for inflammatory bowel disease or colorectal cancer but that persistent symptoms merit prompt investigation (Jones & Rubin, 2009).

Red Flags would be:
- prolonged symptoms
- weight loss
- blood or pus in the diarrhoea
- prostration
- fever
- shock
- recent travel abroad
- recent use of antibiotics.

Most general practitioners would not carry out investigations such as stool culture or blood tests unless the diarrhoea is not abating after a week or there is blood in the stool.

Only 2–5% of stool specimens are positive and even if negative the diarrhoea may still be infective e.g. viruses, traveller's diarrhoea (enterotoxic E. coli). For this reason the HPA recommends that stool samples are only required in certain circumstances (HPA, 2010). These include the 'red flag' circumstances.

Blood tests will normally consist of a CRP, ESR or serum viscosity (raised in bacterial gastroenteritis or inflammatory bowel disease), a full blood count, urea and electrolytes and liver function tests.

The actions of Dr Chowdury in 2008 are reasonable although some GPs might have reassessed Alison in the surgery and requested bloods. Presumably Alison did not attend the outpatient appointment because she was better.

When Alison was seen the following year she had already had symptoms for two weeks. Dr Browne recorded a careful history including the fact that Alison had had a similar episode six months earlier. Dr Browne should have measured a temperature, pulse and blood pressure and palpated the abdomen. However at this stage these would have been largely normal and the omission would not have affected outcome.

At this stage Dr Browne's differential diagnosis should have included infective diarrhoea, anxiety/stress, inflammatory bowel disease (in view of the past history) and diverticulitis. Colorectal cancer, Coeliacs Disease and post-infective irritable bowel were other possibilities although the history was rather short. Alison was not noted to have features to suggest hyperthyroidism.

Dr Browne did not record a differential diagnosis. He organized appropriate blood tests although did not request antibody testing for Coeliacs Disease. Some general practitioners would have arranged a stool culture because of a two-week history of diarrhoea but this was not mandatory.

Dr Browne did record 'very stressed' and appears to have considered 'stress' to be a factor. He had not recorded a history that suggested irritable bowel syndrome (NICE, CG61). Irritable bowel syndrome can follow an episode of infective diarrhoea but the duration of the symptoms was too short to attribute the diarrhoea to this.

In hindsight Dr Browne's choice of anti-diarrhoeal was unfortunate because loperamide can exacerbate inflammatory bowel disease and increase the likelihood of toxic megacolon. However, it is a standard treatment and the only thing which might have alerted him was the previous episode of bloody diarrhoea. Overall his actions were reasonable and although he did not examine Alison this would not have affected the outcome of the consultation.

A potential problem for the practice occurred when the results of the blood tests arrived. A CRP of 83 (and viscosity of 1.91) is high and suggests bacterial colitis or inflammatory bowel disease. The result needed to be considered carefully in the light of the previous history of bloody diarrhoea. The latter made it more likely that Alison had inflammatory bowel disease. Many general practitioners would have contacted Alison when the results were received, assessed her symptoms over the phone and arranged for a reasonably prompt review.

It is clear from the record of the Walk in Centre that Alison was quite unwell. Although she was later recorded as 'systemically well' she was initially noted to be 'pale and unwell'. Alison had a three-week history of worsening diarrhoea which was now bloody, and she had lost weight. It is not clear who saw Alison in the Walk in Centre. If she was assessed by a nurse it would have been reasonable for the nurse to ask for an assessment by a doctor. In any event Alison should have had an abdominal examination and should have had blood tests taken. A competent general practitioner would either have arranged urgent blood tests or have sent her to A&E or the on-call medical team. When her inflammatory markers came back significantly raised she would have been admitted.

It would not be possible to defend Dr White's actions. He recorded an inaccurate history and failed to note either the previous episode of bloody diarrhoea or the raised acute phase reactants. Alison must have clearly been unwell. Although a review was planned it was at too great an interval. Any safety netting would have included features that Alison already had. Alison should have been admitted to hospital.

 Legal comment

We are told that Alison has sued three GPs – Dr Chowdury who saw her initially after her holiday in Goa, Dr Browne who saw her six months later, organized blood tests and arranged a review in two weeks and Dr White who saw her for review only two days before her colleague diagnosed severe ulcerative colitis and toxic megacolon. As indicated in the Expert Opinion, it will be difficult to defend the doctors' standard of care.

We are told Alison has also sued the practice. The partners of the practice are jointly and severally liable for the negligence of each other. But most GPs have legal responsibility for their own errors, and will be indemnified by their MDO. Most partnership agreements make it a requirement that a doctor maintains MDO membership, so that the other partners have that reassurance. So if compensation has to be paid, the MDOs for the responsible doctors will pay for their individual liability. Those partners not responsible will not have to contribute to any settlement.

The blood test results should have prompted action. Is this the liability of the practice as a whole? The results should have been viewed by a GP, who should have initialled them. He or she will be responsible for this failure. If the doctor cannot be identified, then the practice as a whole will be held liable.

Dr White's MDO appears to be the most exposed to this claim. He saw Alison two days before her collapse, when she was already seriously ill. Dr White may have a causation defence; in other words, he may be able to prove that intervention would have made no difference to the outcome. His MDO will instruct an expert to consider whether Alison required surgery anyway, regardless of Dr White's negligence and how much worse her outcome was as a result of Dr White's negligence, if at all.

It seems that for some reason Alison has not sued the Walk in Centre. The MDOs involved in this claim may well wish to seek a contribution from the Centre towards any damages.

 Key learning points

Specific to the case
- If a patient with acute diarrhoea is not unwell it is reasonable to give advice and use the 'test of time'. Self-limiting diarrhoea will usually be due to infective gastroenteritis.
- If the diarrhoea does not settle within 7–10 days it is necessary to review the diagnosis of presumed infective gastroenteritis.
- The possibility of inflammatory bowel disease does need to be considered, and blood inflammatory markers measured, if the diarrhoea does not settle within 7–10 days or there are any 'red flags' such as rectal bleeding or weight loss.
- It is worth bearing in mind that exacerbations of inflammatory bowel disease, or initial presentations, can occur with infective agents such as campylobacter etc.

General
- With any condition that is being observed, it is necessary to set a threshold interval at which time, if the condition has not resolved, the diagnosis needs to be reviewed.
- It is good practice to record the 'safety netting' instruction given and the time period specified.

References and further reading

Cumberland P, Sethi D, Roderick PJ, Wheeler JG, Cowden JM, Roberts JA *et al.* (2003) The infectious intestinal disease study of England: a prospective evaluation of symptoms and health care use after an acute episode. *Epidemiol Infect* **130**: 453–60.

Farthing M, Feldman R, Finch R, Fox R, Leen C, Mandal B *et al.* (1996) The management of infective gastroenteritis in adults a consensus statement by an expert panel convened by the British Society for the study of infection. *Journal of Infection* **33**: 143–52.

Herikstad H, Yang S, Van Gilder TJ *et al.* (2002) A population-based estimate of the burden of diarrhoeal illness in the United States: FoodNet, 1996–97. *Epidemiol Infect* **129**: 9–17.

HPA Primary Care Unit and GP Microbiology Laboratory Use Group, in collaboration with GPs, the AMM and other experts (2010) Infectious Diarrhoea.

The role of microbiological examination of faeces. Quick Reference Guide for Primary Care. For consultation and local adaptation. Produced December 2007 Amended July 2010 following the Griffin Report. Available at http://www.hpa.org.uk/webc/HPAweb File/HPAweb_C/1203582652789

Jones R, Rubin G (2009 Acute diarrhoea in adults. *BMJ* **338**: 46–50.

NICE Guidance CG61: Irritable bowel syndrome in adults: diagnosis and management of irritable bowel syndrome in primary care. http://www.nice.org.uk/CG61.

Wheeler JG, Sethi D, Cowden JM, Wall PG, Rodrigues LC, Tompkins DS *et al.* (1999) Study of infectious intestinal disease in England: rates in the community, presenting to general practice, and reported to national surveillance. The Infectious Intestinal Disease Study Executive. *BMJ* **318**: 1046–50.

Case 9 A young man with back pain

Charlie was 38 and had a long history of back pain and left-sided sciatica. He consulted Dr Mitchell complaining of numbness in the left thigh and buttock for the last 24 hours. Dr Mitchell took a history that excluded any disturbance of sphincter function, and carried out a neurological examination which identified areas of subjective sensory loss in the left L5 dermatome and the S3 dermatome (perianally on the left). There were no other abnormalities on examination. Anal tone was normal. Dr Mitchell rang the local hospital and spoke to an on-call doctor who declined to admit the patient, stating that the clinical picture was not that of cauda equina syndrome; and advised out-patient referral.

The next day Charlie returned to the practice and saw Dr Murphy. He complained of back pain radiating to the right thigh and buttock and down the leg to the hallux. The left-sided sensory symptoms were unchanged. There was no sphincter disturbance. Dr Murphy took the view, based on the record of admission being declined the previous day, that there was still no cauda equina syndrome and that the outpatient referral should be awaited.

A few days later Charlie was admitted to hospital, having developed urinary retention. He had an emergency lumbar decompression of a large disc prolapse that was compressing the cauda equina. The patient brought a claim against both of the GPs, as well as the hospital.

Do you think his claim will succeed?

 ## Expert opinion

Should Dr Mitchell have insisted on admission?

Back pain is extremely common in general practice, accounting for about 10% of consultations. Cauda equina syndrome (CES) is very rare. It usually results from

prolapsed disc material prolapsing centrally rather than laterally (where it just compresses the nerve root at that level).

A GP might on average encounter only one case of CES in a whole career. In this case Dr Mitchell realized that the existence of perianal sensory loss raised the question of cauda equina syndrome and correctly requested a specialist opinion. However, in the absence of other symptoms of cauda equina syndrome most GPs would defer to the advice given by a hospital doctor.

However, the advice received from a nonconsultant grade specialist doctor may not be correct. The distribution of sensory symptoms, particularly if objectively confirmed as signs, is important in the suspicion of CES. The sensory dermatomes are illustrated in Case Figure 9.1.

Bilateral sensory symptoms or signs at the top of the thigh or the lower buttock are suggestive that the cauda equina is involved.

According to Deyo *et al.* (1992) the clinical features that are most likely to predict a cauda equina syndrome are:

1. Disturbance of bladder function;
2. Numbness or paraesthesia in the saddle area; and
3. Numbness at the back of the upper thighs or buttocks (this is the area supplied by the sacral nerves S3 and S4).

Case studies do indicate that 90% of patients with acute cauda equina syndrome have difficulty urinating, However, 75% have disturbance of sensation in the buttocks, posterior upper thighs or perineal region (Deyo *et al.*, 1992). 60% to 80% (not 100%) have reduced anal sphincter tone (Deyo *et al.*, 1992).

Should Dr Murphy have sought admission?

At this point Charlie still had the left-sided perianal sensory disturbance, but now he had right-sided sciatica as well.

Avoiding Errors in General Practice, First Edition. Kevin Barraclough, Jenny du Toit, Jeremy Budd, Joseph E. Raine, Kate Williams and Jonathan Bonser.

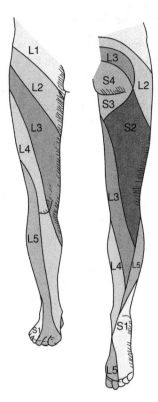

Case Figure 9.1 The sensory dermatomes.

The NICE document *Referral Advice: A Guide to Appropriate Referral from General to Specialist Services* (December 2001) advises that the neurological features suggestive of cauda equina syndrome (and requiring urgent admission) are:

1. '*Sphincter disturbance,*
2. '*Progressive motor weakness,*
3. '*Perineal anaesthesia or*
4. '*Evidence of bilateral nerve root entrapment*'.

Dr Murphy ought to have sought further specialist advice as to the need for admission, because of the new developments overnight.

Legal comment

Cauda equina syndrome is a surprisingly common cause of litigation against GPs, considering its rarity. This must indicate that it is easy to miss. However its effects are very unpleasant and disabling – possibly including permanent urinary and faecal incontinence, need for catheterization, sexual dysfunction, and gait disturbance.

Cases are characterized by disputes of fact as to what symptoms were complained of, and by allegations that urinary symptoms were not properly investigated.

Charlie is suing both the GPs and the hospital. Assuming that the two GPs have different MDOs, each of these three defendants will have separate legal advice. The solicitors acting for each will obtain an expert report on their client's liability.

Dr Murphy's lawyer is the most likely to get unsupportive reports in terms of breach of duty and causation. So he will want to settle the case on the best possible terms. We are not told what the outcome of the surgery was. Charlie may have been left with significant disability. If so, particularly given his age, this could be an expensive claim to settle. Dr Murphy's lawyers (or rather his MDO) will give consideration to whether and to what extent the other two defendants should contribute to a settlement.

Dr Mitchell's lawyer may receive a supportive report. But even that report may be equivocal on whether or not it was negligent for Dr Mitchell to accept the advice of the on-call doctor not to admit Charlie. Dr Mitchell, his MDO and lawyer will then have to give careful consideration to whether they are willing to test the point in Court, or whether they would prefer to contribute to a settlement.

The expert opinion on the on-call doctor's liability will depend to a considerable extent on this doctor's account of what he was told about Charlie's condition. However, Dr Mitchell's detailed note of the conversation will have to be taken into account too. If there are contradictions, then the hospital's lawyers too may be concerned about the risks of proceeding to trial. They may well be willing to discuss contributing to an overall settlement.

It is likely that once each defendant has seen all the evidence and assessed his own strengths and weaknesses, their lawyers will discuss with each other what offer to make to Charlie, and how much each of them should contribute.

As part of this process, Charlie will be asked to submit to a medical examination to assess his current condition and prognosis. The amount offered by the defendants will be based on the findings of that medical examination.

Key learning points

Specific to the case

• The neurological features suggestive of cauda equina syndrome are sphincter disturbance, progressive weakness, perineal anaesthesia and objective signs of bilateral nerve root entrapment.

• Since cauda equina syndrome may develop gradually good records are important not only from the medico-legal point of view, but also to assist later clinicians in assessing what changes may have occurred.

General points
• Good record-keeping is invaluable when defending a case. This includes documenting conversations with secondary care clinicians.
• If there is uncertainty concerning advice from a nonconsultant grade specialist doctor it is worth asking for a second opinion.

References and further reading

Deyo RA, Rainville J, Kent DL (1992) What can the history and physical examination tell us about low back pain? *JAMA* **268**: 760–5.

Lavy C, James A, Wilson-MacDonald J, Fairbank J (2009) Cauda equina syndrome: Clinical Review *BMJ* **338**: b936 doi: 10.1136/bmj.b936.

Case 10 Irregular intermenstrual bleeding in a woman on the pill

Joanna, a 29-year-old housewife, presented to Dr Hanson with a four-month history of intermenstrual bleeding. A year before she had had a normal vaginal delivery of her first baby. Six months ago, when she stopped breast feeding, Joanna changed from the progesterone only pill to the combined contraceptive pill (COCP). Initially she had no problems but for the past four months she had experienced occasional spotting towards the end of the packet.

What would you do?

Joanna had had a normal smear two years ago. Dr Hanson told her that it was common to get breakthrough bleeding on the pill and that it was just a matter of finding a pill that suited. Joanna was given three packets of a different COCP.

She returned a year later to see Dr Bennett. She had had lower abdominal pain and dysuria. She had not continued with the pill because she and her husband wanted to try for another baby. After stopping the COCP her periods had been irregular. She had continued to have intermenstrual and postcoital bleeding but had thought that this was normal after stopping the pill. On examination Joanna did not have a raised temperature. Her lower abdomen was slightly tender. The Dr Bennett did not perform a vaginal examination because Joanna had her period. An MSU was requested and Joanna was given trimethoprim for a presumed urinary tract infection. Dr Bennett informed Joanna that they would let her know if she needed a different antibiotic and also that she should return if she continued to have intermenstrual bleeding.

Would you have done anything differently?

Two months later Joanna returned with continuing symptoms and saw a different partner. Dr Lynch was unable to see the cervix and in view of her persisting symptoms referred Joanna non-urgently to the gynaecologists. Two days later Joanna went to A&E following a heavy postcoital bleed. On examination she was found to have a cervical carcinoma.

Joanna sued the general practitioners on the premise that she should have been examined when she first presented with abnormal vaginal bleeding and that this would have resulted in an earlier diagnosis and treatment on the cervical cancer.

Expert opinion

Cervical cancer is very rare in primary care. The incidence of cervical cancer in the UK fell by 42% between 1988 and 1997 (Peto *et al.*, 2004; Quinn *et al.*, 1999).

A significant problem in general practice is that cancers are rare but symptoms that may signify cancer are very common (Summerton, 2002). Abnormal vaginal bleeding is extremely common in primary care. In one practice in the UK (with 10 000 patients) all women aged 18–54 were sent questionnaires on menstrual problems. In the previous 12 months 25% had experienced menorrhagia, 17% had experienced IMB and 6% PCB (Shapley *et al.*, 2004). It is also recognized that unscheduled bleeding is common during the first three month of using hormonal contraception.

When Joanna first presented it was unlikely that she had cervical cancer. However she had had IMB for four months. The Faculty of Sexual and Reproductive Health recommends that if a woman has unscheduled bleeding on hormonal contraception:
- A clinical history should be taken to determine if there are any associated symptoms and exclude the possibility of a sexually transmitted infection.
- The cervical screening history should be ascertained.
- A pregnancy test should be considered.

If the IMB has been for less than three months and there are no features to suggest a cause other than spotting associated with the hormonal contraception no

Avoiding Errors in General Practice, First Edition. Kevin Barraclough, Jenny du Toit, Jeremy Budd, Joseph E. Raine, Kate Williams and Jonathan Bonser.
© 2013 John Wiley & Sons, Ltd. Published 2013 by John Wiley & Sons, Ltd.

further examination or investigation is required. If however, as in this case, the unscheduled bleeding has been for more than three months a speculum examination should be performed to inspect the cervix (Clinical Effectiveness Unit, 2009). If the cervix had been inspected and was normal it was necessary to ask the patient to return in the middle of the last pill packet in order to check that the IMB had stopped and to prescribe the next supply.

Of menstrual abnormalities (IMB, PCB, menorrhagia) post-coital bleeding (PCB) is the symptom that is probably considered to have the highest likelihood of cervical cancer. One review states: 'Post coital bleeding is regarded as the cardinal symptom of cervical cancer' (Shapley et al., 2006).

A well-constructed systematic review in the British Journal of General Practice, June 2006, examined the likelihood that a woman presenting with post-coital bleeding (PCB) would have cervical cancer (the PPV of the symptom). In the age range 25–34 the chance that a woman presenting with PCB has cervical cancer is estimated at 1 in 5600 (6). This compares with the likelihood that someone aged over 45 with rectal bleeding has colorectal cancer which is likely to be around 5% (Shapley et al., 2006).

There is various and slightly conflicting guidance on indications for specialist referral for women with menstrual bleeding disorders. For PCB referral is variously suggested for 'repeated' (NHS Executive, 2000), 'persistent' (Rosenthal et al., 2001) or 'persistent for more than 4 weeks in women over 35' (NHS Executive, 2000). NICE guidance suggests considering urgent referral for women with persistent IMB and a normal pelvic examination (NICE, 2005). This is particularly the case in women aged over 45 years and, if IMB continues for longer than three months after starting hormonal contraception or there is a change in bleeding pattern in women under 45 years in the presence of risk factors for endometrial carcinoma such as obesity, polycystic ovaries and diabetes.

The place of cervical smears in the investigation of someone with a previously normal cervical smear that has menstrual symptoms is also contentious. A 1997 paper in the British Journal of General Practice made the point that a normal cervical smears does not exclude cervical cancer (because there is a 10% false negative rate) and that IMB and PCB are *not* indicators for a repeat cervical smear (in someone who has previously had a normal smear). 'An additional cervical smear in these circumstances contributes little or nothing to the diagnostic process' (Woodman et al., 1997).

What is clear is that, because cervical smear has a sensitivity of only 80% to 90% for cervical cancer it is not a 'SnOUT'.

The June 2005 NICE guidance advised that abnormal vaginal bleeding should prompt a full pelvic examination with visualization of the cervix. An abnormality of the cervix should prompt referral independent of cervical smear status.

When Joanna presented for the second time Dr Bennett failed to make a full clinical assessment. He/she prematurely anchored on a diagnosis of cystitis and did not consider a differential diagnosis. At this stage it was necessary to: take a good history of the normal pattern of vaginal bleeding, the change in vaginal bleeding, the duration of the change and any co-existent lower genital tract symptoms (such as vaginal discharge, pain on intercourse, PCB); take a history of all drugs that may affect menstrual pattern, particularly the oral contraceptive pill; carry out a pelvic examination, assess the size of the uterus, any adnexal masses, pelvic tenderness and inspect the cervix using a vaginal speculum; take triple swabs. If Joanna had not wanted to be examined because it was her period an appointment should have been made for the following week. At this examination an abnormal cervix would have been seen and an urgent two-week referral made.

 Legal comment

Joanna could name Dr Hanson and Dr Bennett as Defendants in her claim. But she may well decide instead to name the GP practice as a whole.

In principle, a GP partnership (i.e. each individual partner) is liable for the actions not only of their staff but also of each other individual partner. It would usually be a requirement that each medical partner and member of staff has his or her own MDO cover, so that the partnership's liability is met in this way. If for some reason either Dr Hanson or Dr Bennett does not have MDO cover, then the partnership will have to compensate Joanna, and try to then recover the money from the negligent partner (who may or may not have the resources to pay).

In this case, expert opinion suggests that although Dr Hanson may have been negligent (he should have told Joanna to return if the symptoms did not resolve), he may also have a causation defence, i.e. that even if he were negligent, no damage was caused because it is probable that there was no cervical cancer at that time.

Dr Bennett, on the other hand, is in a different position. He should have arranged to do a vaginal examination when he would have made findings leading to an urgent referral. Two months would have been saved.

Would those two months have made a difference to Joanna? That question requires its own expert opinion. If the answer is little or none, then Joanna's compensation will be limited to the extra pain and suffering and distress she has experienced: a few thousand pounds. If it means the difference between life and death, or the loss of her fertility, then this could be a substantial claim.

 Key learning points

Specific to the case

• Cervical cancer is rare in general practice but symptoms that may signify cancer are common.
• Abnormal vaginal bleeding should prompt a full pelvic examination and visualization of the cervix.
• A cervical smear is not an investigation for unexplained vaginal bleeding. Nor is a recent normal smear sufficient reassurance to avoid examination or referral.
• Referral should be considered for persistent PCB and IMB particularly in women over 35 years and 45 years respectively.

General points

• Do not ignore symptoms that do not fit the initial diagnosis. It may be that there is more than one clinical problem to be solved.

References and further reading

Clinical Effectiveness Unit, Royal College of Obstetricians and Gynaecologists (2009) *Faculty of Sexual Health & Reproductive Health Clinical Guidance: Management of Unscheduled Bleeding in Women Using Hormonal Contraception.* May 2009.

Du Toit J, Hamilton W, Barraclough K (2006) Risk in primary care of colorectal cancer from new onset rectal bleeding: 10 year prospective study. *British Medical Journal* **333**: 69-70.

NHS Executive (2000) *Referral Guidelines for Suspected Cancer.* 19-20. London, Department of Health.

NICE (2005) *Referral Guidelines for Suspected Cancer,* CG27.

Peto J, Gilham C, Fletcher O, Matthews FE (2004) The cervical cancer epidemic that screening has prevented in the UK. *The Lancet* **364**: 249–56.

Quinn M, Babb P, Jones J, Allen E (1999) Effect of screening on incidence of and mortality from cancer of cervix in England: evaluation based on routinely collected statistics. *BMJ* **318**: 904.

Rosenthal AN, Panoskaltsis T, Smith T, Soutter WP (2001) The frequency of significant pathology in women attending a general gynaecological service for postcoital bleeding. *British Journal of Obstetrics and Gynaecology* **108**: 103–6.

Shapley M, Jordan K, Croft PR (2004) An epidemiological survey of symptoms of menstrual loss in the community. *British Journal of General Practice* **54**: 359–64.

Shapley M, Jordan K, Croft PR (2006) A systematic review of post coital bleeding and cervical cancer. *British Journal of General Practice* **56**: 453–60.

Summerton N (2002) Symptoms of possible oncological significance: separating the wheat from the chaff. *BMJ* **325**: 1255–6.

Woodman C, Richardson J, Spence M (1997) Why do we continue to take unnecessary cervical smear? *British Journal of General Practice* **47**: 645–6.

Case 11 A boy with a limp

Teddy is 11. He is brought to Dr Hayward by his mother because he has a limp. He was playing football 2 weeks earlier and thinks that he sprained his right knee in a tackle. He is otherwise well with no history of recent illness. On examination he is noted to be obese with a weight of 74 kg. He is apyrexial. He has a slight limp. Dr Hayward notes that Teddy's knee is not swollen but is slightly tender on full flexion.

What is the differential diagnosis and what would you do now?

Dr Hayward diagnoses a knee sprain and advises paracetamol and review in 10 days if the problem has not resolved.

Ten days later the Teddy returns. He is still limping and his pain has not improved. Teddy's right knee seems to be completely normal but Dr Hayward notes that Teddy grimaces when his right hip is fully flexed. Internal rotation is also painful and slightly restricted compared with the left. Dr Hayward requests a FBC, CRP and ESR which are all normal and requests an X-ray of the right hip which is reported as showing no abnormality. She diagnoses a sprained muscle or a transient synovitis and prescribes ibuprofen and arranges to see Teddy again in a month.

Do you agree with the diagnosis? Would you have managed the case differently?

Teddy does not attend the review appointment but then returns three months after the initial visit because he still has a limp and the pain has got significantly worse. Dr Hayward is concerned about the length of time that the limp has lasted for and the degree to which Teddy is limping. She refers him to the paediatric rapid referral clinic where he is seen the next day.

In the paediatric clinic Teddy is apyrexial and is noted to have a limp and a leg that is flexed and externally rotated. There is left hip tenderness and a significantly restricted range of movements. There are no other signs.

The paediatrician asks the radiologist to report the X-rays urgently. The radiologist diagnoses a left-sided slipped upper femoral epiphysis (SUFE) which is clear on the pelvic X-ray and frog leg views.

Teddy's parents bring a case against Dr Hayward alleging that she should have suspected the diagnosis initially and referred him for specialist assessment.

Do you think his claim will succeed?

 ## Expert opinion

A child with a limp is a common occurrence in general practice and causes significant anxiety in both parents and doctors. The problem is commonly due to a minor self limiting condition such as transient synovitis of the hip. However, rarely there is a significant underlying problem and these can be quite easily missed as the initial features may be subtle.

The age of the child determines what serious causes are most likely.

In a child aged under 3, septic arthritis, developmental disorder of the hip or a 'toddler fracture' need to be considered.

In the 3–10 year old, transient synovitis is common but Perthes and septic arthritis also need to be considered.

In the 10–15 year old, a slipped upper femoral epiphysis (SUFE) needs to be considered (particularly in boys), as does Perthes and a septic arthritis.

A slipped upper femoral epiphysis in a teenager is a very rare diagnosis in general practice. However, despite the rarity general practitioners are aware of the diagnosis because of the ease with which the diagnosis can be missed and the potentially serious consequences of late diagnosis. The diagnosis is easily missed

Avoiding Errors in General Practice, First Edition. Kevin Barraclough, Jenny du Toit, Jeremy Budd, Joseph E. Raine, Kate Williams and Jonathan Bonser.
© 2013 John Wiley & Sons, Ltd. Published 2013 by John Wiley & Sons, Ltd.

because the condition is very rare, the symptoms may be mild, and the pain may be in the knee rather than the hip.

A 2004 review in the *BMJ* about the assessment of hip and knee pain notes the following about the differential diagnosis of hip or knee pain in children (Hamer, 2004[1]):

> A child with hip disease may not present with pain or a history of trauma but with an unexplained limp. Unexplained knee pain should raise the suspicion of a hip abnormality ...
>
> Slipped upper femoral epiphysis is typically seen in overweight, hypogonadal boys, who often present with pain referred to the knee, although girls can also be affected. Diagnosis can be difficult, but a 'frog lateral' radiograph will show the deformity. Surgical stabilization is needed urgently to prevent further slippage of the epiphysis ...
>
> Transient synovitis or 'irritable hip' ... [is quite common]

In this case Dr Hayward made several errors which led to a delay in diagnosis. Teddy had a limp and pain in the knee but, as is often the case, the pain was referred from the hip. Teddy grimaced when his knee was flexed because that also involved hip flexion. Once Dr Hayward realized that the problem was in the hip she requested an X-ray but was unaware that a standard AP view is relatively insensitive for detecting SUFE and Perthes. Dr Hayward should have either requested AP and lateral or 'frogs legs' views of both hips or sought urgent specialist assessment.

 Legal comment

Dr Hayward appears to be in breach of her duty of care to Teddy because she did not request the right X-ray views. The next question is what damage did that breach cause? We know that about $2\frac{1}{2}$ months passed before Teddy got the right diagnosis. During that time he certainly suffered pain, for which some (relatively modest) compensation (perhaps £2000–£3000) might be paid. If surgery then completely resolves Teddy's problems, this will be a small claim. But if Teddy is left with some residual

problems, which he would not have had if the diagnosis were made before, then the claim will be more valuable: probably in excess of £100 000. Dr Hayward's legal team will arrange for Teddy to be assessed by an orthopaedic expert who will report on his condition and prognosis. The value of the claim will depend on the findings reported by this expert.

Claims settled on behalf of children are subject to the Court's approval. This is a procedure to make sure the child's interests are properly protected. There will be a hearing at which a District Judge considers all the medical evidence before confirming that the settlement is appropriate.

 Key learning points

Specific to the case
- Remember that hip pain is often referred to the knee.
- The child with the limp is a common presentation in general practice and is commonly due to self limiting disease. However it is necessary to be aware that serious conditions such as SUFE and advanced Perthes can present quite subtly in the well child.

General points
- It is always important to be aware of the limitations of an investigation such as an X-ray.
- Particularly in rare conditions it is advisable to seek specialist advice before interpreting a test as normal if the general practitioner has little experience in the area.

References and further reading

Gough-Palmer A, McHugh K (2007) Investigating hip pain in a well child. *BMJ* **334**: 1216–17.

Hamer A (2004) Pain in the hip and knee. *BMJ* **328**: 1067–9.

Perry DC, Bruce C (2010) Evaluating the child who presents with a limp. *BMJ* **341**: 444–9.

Case 12 A runner with a cough

Fiona consulted Dr Enderby with a three-month history of cough. The cough occurred predominantly on exertion but also sometimes at night and it was not productive. She had not noted shortness of breath particularly, but was training for a marathon and felt her running times were less good than they had been. On direct questioning Dr Enderby established that Fiona had lost a little weight but she was running 60 miles per week in her training. She had also had an eating disorder in the past. Dr Enderby noted that she had a past history of asthma. She was a nonsmoker. Examination was unremarkable, other than that Dr Enderby thought that she looked a little gaunt and underweight. Her PEFR was 500 l/min.

What would you do now?

Dr Enderby treated her for asthma and saw Fiona four times in the next 8 weeks. Initially her symptoms seemed to improve but then she re-presented three months after her initial consultation. Fiona had run her marathon in a reasonable time but felt that, after the initial 'high' following the race her mood had slipped and she had become rather depressed. She was not enjoying her work and was beginning to worry that she would put on weight as she was not running so much. She was not sleeping because she was coughing at night. Dr Enderby started Fiona on fluoxetene and re-started inhaled corticosteroids, which Fiona had stopped. Over the next month her cough improved but her mood deteriorated and she appeared to have lost weight.

What would be your differential diagnosis and how would you discriminate between them?

Dr Enderby was concerned that Fiona was not eating but she stated it was because she was getting heart burn. Dr Enderby referred her to a counsellor specializing in

eating disorders and started her on a PPI. The counsellor found that Fiona's BMI was only 16 and requested a referral to the eating disorders unit, which Dr Enderby did. Fiona was seen three weeks later by a doctor in the eating disorders unit who was concerned that Fiona had a chronic cough and weight loss and requested a chest X-ray. This showed mediastinal lymphadenopathy and Fiona was later diagnosed with stage IIIB Hodgkins disease.

The allegations in the Letter of Claim were that Fiona had had chronic cough for seven months, weight loss for some months and night sweats for two months before diagnosis. It was alleged that Dr Enderby was negligent in that he failed to investigate the cause of the chronic cough, failed to elicit the history of night sweats and failed to monitor Fiona's weight.

Do you think her claim will succeed?

Expert opinion

General practitioners are frequently faced with a patient with many symptoms and many possible causes. In addition mental illness, such as depression or an eating disorder, is a common finding. It is often easy with the benefit of hindsight to see that many of the symptoms were due to a final unifying diagnosis (which is often a relatively rare condition). A chest physician may well be critical of the general practitioner for failing to request a chest X-ray in someone with chronic cough. However, Fiona was a nonsmoker with a history of asthma and many general practitioners would have reasonably considered that the likely differential diagnoses were the 'triad' of asthma, gastro-oesophageal reflux or post-nasal drip syndrome and carried out 'trials of treatment' before requesting a chest X-ray. A general practitioner will not routinely investigate a patient in the way that a specialist will.

Avoiding Errors in General Practice, First Edition. Kevin Barraclough, Jenny du Toit, Jeremy Budd, Joseph E. Raine, Kate Williams and Jonathan Bonser.
© 2013 John Wiley & Sons, Ltd. Published 2013 by John Wiley & Sons, Ltd.

However, a further difficulty about being a generalist is that it is usually necessary to try and integrate disparate bits of information about a patient's history. In this case the allegation was that Dr Enderby was aware of the history of chronic cough and weight loss but, while ascribing them to asthma and an eating disorder, failed to consider the possibility that they may be related. Dr Enderby was criticized for failing to follow up on the history of chronic cough (though it was persisting), failing to consider a differential diagnosis for the weight loss and failing to monitor the weight loss (document the weights) and investigate the same before assuming that it was due to an eating disorder.

This is a type of case that tests the standard required of general practitioners. It is possible that different experts would have different opinions in a case like this. Dr Enderby's actions were not 'careless' in the accepted sense of the word (one of the definitions of breach of duty). At each stage he had a plausible diagnosis and acted appropriately for that diagnosis.

However, the standard required diagnostically is likely to be quite high for a well-paid and highly trained professional. In this case Fiona had a long history of illness and Dr Enderby's actions suggest that he did not fully consider the differential diagnoses that were necessary to be considered. He appears to have prematurely anchored on two diagnoses and failed to reconsider these when treatment failed and the initial presentation evolved. My own opinion is that Dr Enderby was in breach of duty once a reasonable therapeutic trial for chronic cough had failed and once it became apparent that the (undocumented) weight loss was a significant factor to be carefully considered.

 Legal comment

Expert opinion suggests that Dr Enderby's actions or omissions are at the very edge of what may be considered acceptable practice. The expert says his own opinion is that Dr Enderby was in breach of duty at a certain point in this scenario. While an expert may have his own opinion, what is important is whether there is a responsible body of medical opinion (even if it is not the expert's) that would support Dr Enderby's actions. Maybe there is. If so, how sound are the reasons for this opinion?

Some difficult judgements will have to be made by Dr Enderby and his legal team. Should the case be defended to trial or should they settle? Generally, the MDOs take cases to trial that receive strong supportive opinions. After all, if the case is lost, not only will Dr Enderby's reputation suffer but also a judicial precedent may be set which makes life harder for other doctors. Furthermore, defending this case to trial could cost the MDO several tens of thousands of pounds.

The MDO will also take into account the likely value of the claim. This will depend on the causation and condition and prognosis evidence that they receive. If the claim is of modest value, then the reluctance to take the risk will probably be all the greater.

 Key learning points

Specific to the case
- Chronic cough in a nonsmoker who is not taking ACE inhibitors is usually one of the triad: asthma, gastroesophageal reflux or post-nasal drip syndrome.
- However, treatment failure or features that 'do not fit' such as weight loss should prompt investigation.
- There should be a low threshold for carrying out a chest X-ray in chronic cough;

General point
- It is often difficult in general practice keep track of all the threads of multiple symptoms

Further reading

Barraclough K (2009) Diagnosis in general practice: chronic cough in adults, *BMJ* **338**: b1218, doi: 10.1136/bmj.b1218.

Case 13 A woman with classical migraine

Rachel consulted Dr Dewan. She was aged 48 and stated that she had suffered from migraines all her life. She had never previously sought medical advice about the matter. In the last month she had had three episodes of severe left sided headache associated with visual disturbance in her left eye. She thought that the lights at work (she worked in a call centre) triggered the attacks because she had twice experienced them when leaving work. She had vomited once.

What would you do now? What bits of information would you want to elicit?

Dr Dewan took Rachel's blood pressure and checked that her fundi were normal. She suggested a trial of a triptan wafer, which would be absorbed through the buccal mucosa and thus would be absorbed even if Rachel was nauseated.

Ten days later Rachel consulted the Out of Hours service with a severe left-sided unilateral headache, vomiting and visual disturbance. She was given an injection of an intramuscular opiate and prochlor-perazine.

On the following Monday Rachel consulted Dr Dewan again. Her symptoms had all resolved but she was concerned at the frequency of the migraine attacks and the visual disturbances which were new to her. Dr Dewan suggested that she try propanolol to reduce the frequency and severity of the attacks.

Three days later Rachel consulted one of Dr Dewan's colleagues. He was experiencing another migraine and she stated that the vision in her right eye was blurred. The doctor noted that her right eye was slightly red, measured her blood pressure, noted he could not visualize the fundus, and questioned the diagnosis of cluster headaches. He referred her for a neurological opinion. He also advised that she see an optician to measure the pressure in her eyes.

What would be your differential diagnosis and how would you discriminate between them?

The following day Rachel attended the surgery again as an emergency. She had been vomiting overnight, had a red right eye, reduced visual acuity and had perception of light only in that eye. The doctor referred her immediately to hospital and she was diagnosed with acute angle closure glaucoma. The ophthalmology SHO noted a history of recurrent episodes of uniocular blurring of vision, visual haloes and that these had occurred twice when she left work (she worked nights at a call centre). She was treated but was left with perception of light only in her right eye.

Rachel made a claim against the practice alleging that if Dr Dewan had taken a careful history it would have been clear that her new visual symptoms were uniocular rather than homonymous.

Do you think her claim will succeed?

 Expert comment

General practitioners have relatively little training in, or experience of, significant eye disease. Training in ophthalmology usually comprises a couple of weeks as a medical student and an occasional day course in ophthalmology once qualified.

Despite this, it is relatively common for general practitioners to be consulted about visual symptoms and 'the red eye'.

The most important aspects of assessing visual disturbances is to establish whether the visual disturbance is in both eyes and extends over the visual field (placing the disturbance behind the optic chiasm and most likely in the occipital cortex) or in one eye (placing the disturbance most likely in the eye itself). If the disturbance

Avoiding Errors in General Practice, First Edition. Kevin Barraclough, Jenny du Toit, Jeremy Budd, Joseph E. Raine, Kate Williams and Jonathan Bonser.

is in one eye it is important to check whether there is any pain, whether the eye is red or not, measure a visual acuity and look at the fundus.

If the visual disturbance is transient and homonymous (affecting the visual field rather than one eye) then the diagnosis is very likely to be a migrainous aura. Typically the patient will describe shimmering, often coloured lights, it may be difficult but not impossible to see through the visual obscuration (sometimes described like a fog) and the negative scotoma may migrate slowly over the visual field and resolve after 10 to 30 minutes.

If, on the other hand, the visual disturbance is in one eye it will be likely that the cause is pathology in that eye. Migraine can be associated with uniocular (retinal) auras but it is very rare. Uniocular flashing lights or scintillating spectra or scotomas are much more likely to be due to retinal tears or detachments. Uniocular flashing lights usually indicate vitreoretinal traction caused by a posterior vitreous detachment.

Uniocular visual blurring with haloes around bright lights (similar to those that occur on a window wet with condensation) is very likely to be due to corneal oedema from a acute angle closure glaucoma. This is particularly the case if there is a unilateral red eye, headache or vomiting.

Ophthalmological conditions do pose a problem for general practitioners because of the lack of expertise and the lack of specialized equipment. However, a few basic rules can ensure that serious conditions are unlikely to be missed:

1. Always establish if any visual symptoms are uniocular or binocular, and whether they are transient or persistent (if bilateral the problem is in the brain).
2. Always check for a red eye and ask about pain (iritis, acute glaucoma and conjunctivitis).
3. It is usually necessary to measure a visual acuity (see below).
4. Always check that the pupils are round and responsive to light (irregular or fixed in iritis and acute glaucoma).

If there is visual disturbance it is also useful to establish if straight lines are distorted (wet macular degeneration). If there is a localized area of loss of vision in one eye (a scotoma) it is useful to check whether it is a positive scotoma (something obscuring vision) or a negative scotoma (like the 'blind spot' in the eye). A positive scotoma is usually due to something in front of the retina like a detachment flopping in front, a vit-

reous bleed or a vitreous floater. A negative scotoma is usually due to a retinal problem (chronic simple glaucoma or a retinal infarction) or a brain problem (such as a stroke).

Visual acuity should be measured with a retro illuminated Snellen chart, with and without a pinhole. The Snellen chart pinned onto the wall with Blu-tack suffers from the problem that the contrast between the black letters and the background is low, so the elderly with slight cataracts will have poor acuity despite having no significant pathology. The pinhole acts like a pinhole camera and largely corrects for any refractive error. This is something that is not widely utilized among non-ophthalmologists.

In this case there were a number of problems which are relatively common in medico-legal cases involving visual symptoms.

Rachel's visual symptoms were clearly uniocular from the start. As such they were very unlikely to be due to migraine. Once she had a red eye it was most unlikely that her red eye was due to cluster headaches. It was much more likely that she was getting episodes of angle closure glaucoma when she walked from the brightly lit call centre (with a contracted pupil) to the dark night (with a large pupil obstructing the drainage angle).

Dr Dewan appears to have mixed up chronic simple glaucoma (in which case opticians often measure chronically elevated intra ocular pressures) and acute angle closure glaucoma (which is an ophthalmological emergency and when the intraocular pressure may be normal between episodes).

The final doctor should have realized that one of the purposes of using an ophthalmoscope is to test the clarity of the media in the eye. If the doctor cannot look in and see the retina the patient probably cannot look out.

 Legal comment

It seems that Rachel has lost nearly all the sight of one eye because Dr Dewan and his colleagues failed to recognize an ophthalmological emergency. Clearly, the case will have to be settled. The loss of sight in one eye will be worth in the region of £35 000. Rachel may well have suffered other losses which should also be compensated, e.g. cost of any special aids she may need to help her through the rest of her life. She will also have a claim for any psychological effects that she may suffer.

Key learning points

Specific to the case

• Ophthalomogical problems are relatively common causes of cases against general practitioners. They missed conditions are usually iritis, acute angle closure glaucoma or retinal detachments.

• General practitioners have difficulties with such cases. However, one is unlikely to miss anything with 4 basic rules:

1. Always establish if any visual symptoms are uniocular or binocular, and whether they are transient or persistent (if bilateral the problem is in the brain).
2. Always check for a red eye and ask about pain (iritis, acute glaucoma and conjunctivitis).
3. It is usually necessary to measure a visual acuity (see below).
4. Always check that the pupils are round and responsive to light (irregular or fixed in iritis and acute glaucoma).

• Visual acuity should ideally be measured with a retro illuminated Snellen chart with and without a pinhole.

General points

• With many diagnoses in general practice (and ophthalmological diagnoses are a good example) a careful history together with a very focused examination will exclude the possibility of significant disease.

Further reading

Bal SK, Hollingworth GR (2005) The 'Red eye', *BMJ* **331**: 438.

Wilson J (2010) Eye emergencies, *InnovAiT* **3**: 509–17.

Case 14 A young woman with diarrhoea and vomiting

Martha was 30 when she saw Dr Vickers, an out-of-hours general practitioner, with a four-hour history of upper abdominal pain followed by vomiting. Dr Vickers recorded there had been indigestion earlier and the pain had moved down. On examination there was some abdominal tenderness (site not recorded). Dr Vickers prescribed some ranitidine. No follow-up advice was recorded.

Martha sought further Out of Hours advice 48 hours later from Dr Clelland, giving a history of severe abdominal pain and fever. The antacid had helped but the pain had returned. Dr Clelland thought the symptoms consistent with gastritis.

Two days later Martha had a laparotomy for a perforated appendix with peritonitis (which had been present for some time).

Why was the diagnosis of appendicitis missed?

 ## Expert comment

Acute abdominal pain is a very common reason for consultations in primary care. The possible causes are legion. In the majority of cases general practitioners are trying to differentiate between those patients who may have a 'surgical' acute abdomen and the vast majority who are suffering from self limiting causes of abdominal pain. The incidence of acute abdominal pain presenting to general practitioners or A&E departments is quoted as 11 to 13 per 1000 patients per year (de Wit, 2004). Of these many will be self-limiting conditions that can be managed in the community and observed. A full-time general practitioner will therefore expect to see one or two patients a month with acute abdominal pain.

Appendicitis is a common cause of a surgical acute abdomen and is a frequent cause of litigation against GPs when it is missed and goes on to cause perforation and/ or peritonitis.

For reasons that are not quite clear the incidence of acute appendicitis has been falling for some decades. The quoted incidence of acute appendicitis in the Western world is between 0.7 and 1.6 per 1000 per year (de Wit, 2004). This suggests that a general practitioner may see 1 to 2 cases on his/her list per year. However, in practice a fulltime general practitioner probably now only sees a case of acute appendicitis once every couple of years or so.

The presentation of acute appendicitis is often rather atypical. The variation in the types of clinical presentation of acute appendicitis is often attributed to the anatomical site of the inflamed appendix (since Sir Zachary Cope's classical work on *The early diagnosis of the acute abdomen* in 1921 (Cope, 1921). A clinical presentation of acute appendicitis with diarrhoea is a recognized cause of diagnostic error and delay (Murch, 2000).

However at the first consultation in this case the following features were present:
- acute onset of abdominal pain; some vomiting;
- pain starting high and moving down;
- pain on abdominal palpation;
- low-grade fever.

On the face of it these symptoms and signs seem to tally quite well with the 'classical' presentation of appendicitis; a history over a few days of generalized central or lower abdominal pain, migrating to the right iliac fossa (as the peritoneal surfaces over the inflamed appendix also become inflamed), with vomiting, constipation and a slightly raised temperature (Wagner *et al.*, 1996).

A review article in the *Journal of the America Medical Association* considers the sensitivity and specificity of history features and examination findings for appendicitis (Wagner *et al.*, 1996). The article shows that the presence or absence of right lower quadrant pain/tenderness is highly discriminatory, and other features such as the migration of the pain from the centre of the abdomen to the right lower quadrant, pain before vomiting, rigidity and guarding are also very helpful.

Avoiding Errors in General Practice, First Edition. Kevin Barraclough, Jenny du Toit, Jeremy Budd, Joseph E. Raine, Kate Williams and Jonathan Bonser.
© 2013 John Wiley & Sons, Ltd. Published 2013 by John Wiley & Sons, Ltd.

In this case the appendicitis was missed. Dr Vickers saw Martha early in the course of her illness. It would have been helpful if he/she had taken a slightly more detailed history and recorded the site of the abdominal tenderness. His/her actions might have been reasonable if careful safety netting advice has been given and recorded.

The consultation demonstrates the cognitive errors of 'premature anchoring' – a reluctance to depart from a mundane diagnosis such as gastroenteritis, which the doctor may have seen fairly frequently and 'premature diagnostic closure' – in other words a reluctance to obtain or consider further information that may cast doubt on the first diagnostic hypothesis.

At the second consultation Dr Clelland may have been unduly influenced by the prescription of ranitidine by the first GP, leading to a diagnosis of gastritis despite the complaints of severe pain and lower abdominal pain. If he/she had examined Martha's abdomen it is likely that she would have had guarding or rebound in the right iliac fossa. If no examination was done Dr Clelland was in breach of duty.

This consultation demonstrates 'confirmation bias', leading a doctor to prefer to elicit or favour clinical data that supports the chosen hypothesis (e.g. the report that the ranitidine tablets had helped) rather than the date inconsistent with it (e.g. that the pain was now lower abdominal).

If no definite diagnosis can be made, it is prudent to follow the patient up soon, in order to judge whether the symptoms are changing. It can be very helpful to such follow-up if some basic blood tests are obtained. It is also necessary to give and document careful safety netting advice.

In the same general category as the case above is the misdiagnosis of acute gastroenteritis. This illness would typically involve the onset of nausea and vomiting lasting for some hours (up to 24) followed by diarrhoea, which might persist for some days. Abdominal pain is usually colicky, not localized, and usually precedes an episode of diarrhoea. This 'classical' picture can lead to a confident diagnosis of gastroenteritis.

When gastroenteritis is diagnosed in the face of persisting vomiting; continuous or localized pain; and in the absence of diarrhoea; the GP is vulnerable to the allegation of having made an untenable diagnosis and therefore having closed his or her mind to the alternatives.

 Legal comment

Both Dr Vickers and Dr Clelland seem each to have negligently failed to consider a possible diagnosis of appendicitis. If the correct diagnosis had been made, it is probable that perforation and peritonitis could have been avoided.

Martha therefore appears to have a good claim for compensation for the pain and suffering caused by the perforation and peritonitis. This may only be a few thousand pounds (depending on the circumstances). However, if the peritonitis has caused lasting consequences, then they too would be the subject of compensation. For example, if her fertility is compromised, as a young woman she may have a right to compensation of several tens of thousands of pounds.

 Key learning points

Specific to the case
- Do ask about the onset and time course of the illness (particularly vomiting, pain, and diarrhoea).
- Do not rely on a diagnosis of gastritis or gastroenteritis in patients with prolonged symptoms, atypical symptoms, or severe pain.
- Do follow up any patient with atypical symptoms or localized pain. It is always wise to review the patient with acute abdominal pain the next day.

General point
- An awareness of the cognitive errors of premature anchoring, premature diagnostic closure and confirmation bias helps to avoid diagnostic errors.

References and further reading

Cope Z (1921) *The Early Diagnosis of the Acute Abdomen.* Oxford University Press.

de Wit N (2004) Acute abdominal pain. In R Jones, N Britten, L Culpepper *et al.* (eds), *Oxford Textbook of Primary Medical Care*, pp. 738–42. Oxford University Press.

Murch S (2000) Diarrhoea, diagnostic delay and appendicitis. *The Lancet* **356**: 787.

Wagner JM, McKinney WP, Carpenter JL (1996) Does this patient have appendicitis? *Journal of the American Medical Association* **276**: 1589–93.

Case 15 Ill-fitting dentures in an elderly man

Alfred was a 74-year-old man with previously good health who rarely attended the surgery. He consulted Dr McDowd with a two-week history of 'flulike' symptoms, fever, sinusitis and lack of appetite. He had lost a little weight but he attributed that to problems he was having with his dentures. Dr McDowd found that Alfred was apyrexial with a clear chest and prescribed amoxicillin.

Eight days later Alfred consulted Dr McDowd again. He felt a little better but his wife was concerned that he had lost some more weight. He was seeing his dentist because his lower denture was causing him pain, which inhibited him from eating. His fever had gone but he still had sinus pain. Dr McDowd found a temperature of 37.4 C and a normal pulse and blood pressure. He prescribed doxycycline.

What would you do now?

Three days later Alfred's wife telephoned Dr McDowd and explained that she was worried about her husband. He was not eating, was not himself and the problems with his dentures were 'getting him down'. She wondered if he had an infection in his sinuses. Dr McDowd arranged some blood tests and sinus X-rays.

The following day Alfred saw Dr Elsworth at the practice. He explained that he had picked up an infection a few weeks ago and had been 'unable to shift it'. He was wondering about another antibiotic. Dr Elsworth noted that Alfred had malaise, weight loss, generalized aches and pains and sinusitis. He noted that Alfred had not had the blood tests or sinus X-rays. He rang the radiology department and was informed that they no longer did sinus X-rays at the request of general practitioners. He prescribed some clarithromycin and a nasal decongestant.

The following day Dr McDowd received the blood test results. Alfred had a CRP of 70 mg/l and an ESR of 64 mm/hr. His full blood count showed an anaemia of 10.9 g/dl with a normal MCV. Dr McDowd also received a form from an optician stating that Mr McDowd had had intermittent double vision but that examination was normal. Dr McDowd requested a serum ferritin, B12 and folate and a fasting blood glucose.

What would be your differential diagnosis and how would you discriminate between them?

The following day Alfred rang Dr McDowd and told him that he could had woken unable to see out of his left eye. Dr McDowd advised him to go straight to A&E. The A&E SHO elicited a history of jaw claudication and bi temporal headache and impalpable temporal arteries. A diagnosis of giant cell arteritis was made. Alfred was admitted and started on high dose methyl prednisolone but did not regain the sight in his left eye.

A claim was brought against Dr McDowd and Dr Elsworth that they should have suspected that Alfred could have giant cell arteritis, started him on high dose corticosteroids and referred him.

Do you think his claim will succeed?

 Expert comment

Headaches and facial pain are extremely common presentations in general practice and patients often self diagnose acute sinusitis incorrectly (Murtagh, 2004). Most patients with acute sinusitis will have objective fever and a purulent nasal discharge as well as facial pain or headache (Williams & Simel, 1993). Acute sinusitis is comparatively unlikely unless all three are present.

Avoiding Errors in General Practice, First Edition. Kevin Barraclough, Jenny du Toit, Jeremy Budd, Joseph E. Raine, Kate Williams and Jonathan Bonser.
© 2013 John Wiley & Sons, Ltd. Published 2013 by John Wiley & Sons, Ltd.

General practitioners need to be extremely cautious with the assessment of headaches in the older patient. The commonest causes of headaches, tension headaches and migraine, are not common in the elderly. Giant cell arteritis is not particularly rare in this age group and a full-time general practitioner will see a new case every couple of years. The presentation is often atypical with typical temporal headache being absent in nearly 50% of patients. Patients with ischaemic symptoms (jaw claudication and/or visual disturbances, including diplopia) are at high risk of sudden visual loss (Slavarni *et al.*, 2005). Yet these patients (and the patients with predominantly systemic symptoms of weight loss, fever, myalgia and malaise) are the most likely to be missed by doctors (Ezeonyeji *et al.*, 2011).

In this case both Dr McDowd and Dr Elsworth did not pick up on several clues: malaise and weight loss in a 74 year old is usually not due to mild self-limiting disease. Facial pain due to acute sinusitis is uncommon in this age group. Alfred effectively had high inflammatory markers that were not otherwise explained. A new history of multiple consultations together with expressions of concern from a spouse is often an indicator of serious disease in an elderly person. However, the main problem appears to have been that the general practitioners were not sufficiently aware of the protean manifestations of GCA and the requirement of a very high index of suspicion to avoid missing the diagnosis. A 2002 systemic review analyzed 1435 cases of GCA. The mean duration of symptoms by the time of diagnosis was 3.5 months. Case Table 15.1 indicates the protean manifestations of the condition (Smetana & Shmerling, 2002),

Case Table 15.1 Protean manifestations of GCA.

Clinical feature	Percentage of biopsy proven cases with the feature (sensitivity)
Temporal headache	52
Any headache	76
Scalp tenderness	31
Jaw claudication	34
Any visual symptom	37
Unilateral visual loss	24
Diplopia	9
Myalgia	39
Previous diagnosis of PMR	34
Weight loss	43
Fever	42
Absent temporal pulse	45
Any abnormality on palpation of the temporal artery (absent, prominent, beaded)	65
ESR 'normal'	4
ESR > 50	83

require extra care as a result of his lost vision in the left eye.

 Legal comment

Neither Dr McDowd nor Dr Elsworthy recognized that they were dealing with a number of high inflammatory markers which needed an explanation. If high dose cortico-steriods had been prescribed sooner and an urgent referral had been made would the sight in Alfred's left eye have been saved?

A GP expert will have to analyze the case in retrospect to identify the point at which Alfred should have been recognized as an emergency. Then an ophthalmologist will have to assess whether an urgent referral at that point would probably have saved the sight in Alfred's left eye. If the answer is yes, probably, then compensation will have to be paid to Alfred. The compensation for his pain and suffering is likely to be in the region of £35 000. Alfred may be able to claim further damages, if he will

 Key learning points

Specific to the case
- Unless a patient has all three features of acute sinusitis (fever, facial pain and purulent nasal discharge) the diagnosis is unlikely to be correct.
- 50% of cases of GCA do not present with typical temporal headaches.
- Many patients present with non specific systemic symptoms of malaise, myalgia, fever and weight loss.
- Ischaemic symptoms (jaw claudication or visual symptoms) are associated with a high risk of visual loss.
- If there is any reason to suspect GCA it is necessary to start high dose oral corticosteroids (60 mg of prednisolone daily) immediately

References and further reading

Ezeonyeji A, Borg F, Dasgupta B (2011) Delays in recognition and management of giant cell arteritis: results from a retrospective audit. *Clinical Rheumatology* **30**: 259–62.

Hassan N, Dasgupta B, Barraclough K (2011) Easily missed?: Giant cell arteritis *BMJ* **342**: 1201–1206. doi:10.1136/bmj.d3019.

McMinn J, Steel C, Bowman A (2011) Investigation and management of unintentional weight loss in older adults. *BMJ* **342**: 754–9.

Murtagh J (2004) Headache and facial pain. In In R Jones, N Britten, L Culpepper *et al.* (eds), *Oxford Textbook of Primary Medical Care*, pp. 1045–9. Oxford University Press.

Slavarni C, Cimino L, Macchioni P, *et al.* (2005) Risk factors for visual loss in an Italian population-based cohort of patients with giant cell arteritis. *Arthritis Rheum* **53**: 293–7.

Smetana GW, Shmerling RH (2002) Does this patient have temporal arteritis? *JAMA* **287**: 92–101.

Williams JW, Simel DL (1993) Does this patient have sinusitis? *JAMA* **270**: 1242–6.

Case 16 Back pain in a middle-aged woman

Angela had been registered at the practice for three years when she consulted Dr Ahmed about her back pain. She had initially become aware of lumbar ache four months earlier, after helping her daughter move into a new flat. The pain was just to the right of the lower thoracic spine with no radiation. Initially the pain had been relieved by ibuprofen or paracetamol but more recently the pain was more persistent and was disturbing her sleep somewhat. She was otherwise well.

What would you do now? Are any particular features on examination likely to be helpful?

Dr Ahmed found that Angela had a full range of movement of the spine and straight leg raising was symmetric and unimpeded. Spinal percussion was not painful.

Dr Ahemd prescribed some co-codamol, advised Angela to keep mobile and suggested she return if the pain was no better in one month.

A month later Angela returned and the pain was no better. She described the pain as being slightly lower down the back by this time, and she had pain radiating into her right anterior thigh which kept her awake at night.

What would be your differential diagnosis and how would you discriminate between them?

Dr Ahmed found that there was no weakness of hip flexion or knee flexion and extension but that right ankle dorsiflexion was weak and the right knee reflex was absent. He wondered about a lumbar disc prolapse but decided to obtain blood tests (FBC, ESR, CRP, U + E and LFTs) and obtain X-rays of the lumbar spine.

The ESR was 28 but otherwise the blood tests were largely normal. However, the X-ray was reported as showing a bone cyst in the third lumbar vertebra and

the radiologist's report suggested a myeloma screen. Dr Ahmed asked the receptionists to ask Angela to make an appointment for a blood and urine test. He was then on holiday for two weeks. The myeloma screen was seen by one of his colleagues and was negative.

Three months later Angela returned to see one of Dr Ahmed's colleagues. She was in a great deal of pain and had lost some weight. Her right leg was weak and she had difficulty passing urine. She was admitted to hospital and found to have a large vertebral metastasis affecting L3 and L4 and cord compression. It was noted in hospital that she had a history of breast cancer treated successfully 18 years earlier. This information was in the general practice correspondence but was not on the computerized summary. She underwent emergency radiotherapy but was left with urinary incontinence and weakness of her right leg.

Angela brought a claim against Dr Ahmed alleging that he should have considered her past history of breast cancer, her night pain and her age and referred her for urgent specialist care. It was further alleged that the lumbar spine X-ray results had not been acted upon.

Do you think her claim will succeed?

 Expert comment

Back pain is extremely common in the general population and is an extremely common complaint in general practice. The annual incidence of significant back pain is estimated at 5% and the point prevalence in the population at 25%. Most back pain is benign and self-limiting. 90% of people will have substantially improved by 6 weeks from the onset.

In primary care approximately 0.7% of patients presenting with back pain have metastatic cancer, 4% have osteoporotic stress fractures, 0.3% have ankylosing spondylitis and 0.01% have spinal infections (Deyo et al., 1992; Jarvik & Deyp, 2002).

Avoiding Errors in General Practice, First Edition. Kevin Barraclough, Jenny du Toit, Jeremy Budd, Joseph E. Raine, Kate Williams and Jonathan Bonser.

The 1999 guidance document produced by the Royal College of General Practitioners listed the following 'red flags' (with referral guidance):

Red flags for *possible* serious spinal pathology:
- Presentation under age 20 or onset over 55
- Non-mechanical pain
- Thoracic pain
- Past history - carcinoma, steroids, HIV
- Unwell, weight loss
- Widespread neurological symptoms or signs
- Structural deformity

The difficulty is that not all these 'red flags' are equal. Studies show that some, such as age over 55, nonmechanical back pain and thoracic back pain, make up a significant proportion of the population consulting in primary care and are not particularly helpful for identifying rare cases of cancer or infection. Most studies indicate that back pain is not relieved at night by lying down in nearly half of all patients with simple mechanical back pain (Deyo *et al.*, 1992; Van den Hoogen *et al.*, 1995). Nearly a sixth of people consulting have thoracic pain and one-third to one-quarter are aged over 55 (Deyo *et al.*, 1992; Van den Hoogen *et al.*, 1995).

However, a history of cancer, particularly those cancers that tend to metastasize to bone (such as breast, colon, prostate, lung, renal) has a very high likelihood that the back pain will be due to metastases. In one study of 1975 patients presenting in primary care 13 had bone metastases. Out of the 1975 only 45 had a history of cancer and 4 (9%) had vertebral metastases causing their back pain (Deyo *et al.*, 1992). Other studies also suggest that about 10% for of those with back and a history of cancer will have bone metastases.

Spinal tenderness to percussion is equally common in patients with and without cancer and is unhelpful.

An ESR of over 20 mm/hr occurs in about 80% of patients with vertebral metastases. However, the usefulness of the test is limited by the fact that about a third of patients without cancer have an ESR over 20 (the specificity is low at about 65%). 70% of patients with vertebral metastases have X-ray changes (lytic or sclerotic lesions or crush fractures). Virtually no patients without cancer or a vertebral crush fracture will have these clinical features, making an X-ray reasonably discriminatory though isotope bone scans are obviously much more sensitive.

This case does illustrate several problems that are not uncommon in medico-legal cases.

It is clinically unsafe if significant past medical events are not recorded in a prominent position in computerized notes. In this case the past history of treated breast cancer was clear in the correspondence, but when the notes were being summarized for the computer when Angela registered at the practice the history was not recorded on the summary. This can lead to very serious clinical oversights, as in this case. A junior doctor seeing a patient for the first time in hospital will usually ask the patient about their past medical history. A general practitioner rarely does this in a 10-minute consultation if there appears to be a complete summary on the computer.

A second relatively common problem occurs when another general practitioner sees a normal result, is not familiar with the patient but assumes that, because the result is normal (the myeloma screen in this case) no further action is necessary. It is understandable that the colleague checking Dr Ahmed's results does not scrutinize the history with all normal blood results. However, Dr Ahmed needed to alert the colleague covering in his absence that Angela had a lytic bone lesion, and that further action was required.

A third problem is that general practitioners are not used to looking at or interpreting X-rays. As such they rely heavily on the radiologist's report. In this case an expert radiologist was critical of the standard of the radiology report. It did not make it clear to the general practitioner that the differential diagnosis of the lytic bone lesion included things other than myeloma. However, it was reasonable to expect a general practitioner to know this.

Dr Ahmed had considered that the likely pathology was a disc prolapse affecting the right L4 nerve (and causing the loss of the knee reflex). However, disc prolapses other than L5/S1 or L4/L5 are rather unusual and, particularly in the older patient, should but the general practitioner on alert that the radiculopathy may be due to malignant disease.

The case was clearly indefensible on breach of duty. The practice as a whole was liable for the poor quality of the computerized notes and Dr Ahmed was liable for failing to act in the light of the past history of cancer and failing to act properly on the radiology report. The case illustrates how medical errors normally only occur when several things go wrong sequentially.

 Legal comment

Expert opinion is clear that there has been a breach of duty by Dr Ahmed. It seems that from the start he should have had the possibility in mind of a metastasis. As it was, the diagnosis was made about four months late. If Angela had had radiotherapy four months sooner, what would the outcome have been on the balance of probabilities? Would she have had urinary incontinence and/or weakness of the right leg?

Angela's lawyers and Dr Ahmed's lawyers will each obtain an expert opinion on these causation questions. They may well arrange for these two experts to meet to discuss the case, and see if they can come to a common view. If they conclude that earlier treatment would have saved Angela from the leg weakness and incontinence, the lawyers will start to negotiate a settlement.

It may be possible to obtain a contribution towards the settlement from the hospital in relation to the poor quality of the X-ray report. If the practice is comprised of partners who belong to a different MDO from that of Dr Ahmed, then his MDO may also ask for a contribution from them in relation to the practice's failure to keep proper computerized records. However, these contributions are not likely to be significant.

 Key learning points

Specific to the case

• A past history of cancer carries with it about a 10% risk that a new episode of back pain will be due to cancer. It has a far higher predictive value of cancer than other 'Red Flags' such as non mechanical pain, age over 55 or thoracic pain.

• Tenderness on spinal percussion does not discriminate between cancer and benign disease.
• It is important to be aware of the rough radiological differential diagnosis of common findings.

General points

• It is very important within the context of short consultations in general practice that a patient's significant past medical history is well summarized.
• Errors can occur when a colleague is interpreting clinical results without knowledge of the context of the test.

References and further reading

Deyo RA, Rainville J, Kent DL (1992) What can the history and physical examination tell us about low back pain? *JAMA* **268**: 760–5.

Jarvik J, Deyp R (2002) Diagnostic evaluation of low back pain with emphasis on imaging. *Annals of Internal Medicine* **137**: 586–97.

Van den Hoogen HM, Koes BW, van Eijk JT, Bouter LM (1995) On the accuracy of history, physical examination and erythrocyte sedimentation rate in diagnosing low back pain in general practice: a criteria based review of the literature. *Spine* **22**: 318–27.

Case 17 Cellulitis in a man's foot

Reg was an overweight 76-year-old retired shopkeeper who consulted Dr Berg in an emergency appointment with a three-day history of a painful left foot. He was taking bendroflumethiazide for hypertension, had a previous history of gout and was an ex-smoker. On examination the left forefoot was red and swollen. Dr Berg diagnosed cellulitis and treated Reg with flucloxacillin.

Would you have done anything differently?

Three days later Reg returned to see a different doctor because of continuing pain. Dr Haynes recorded that the foot was numb as well as painful. The foot was still red. Dr Haynes diagnosed gout, checked a uric acid level and treated Reg with diclofenac. When the blood result returned the urate level was just above normal. Dr Haynes felt that this confirmed her diagnosis and she did not contact the patient.

Would this result have reassured you?

Reg requested a visit four days later when the pain in his foot was so bad that he could not get out of bed. His left foot was a dusky blue and became pale when elevated. It did not feel particularly cold. However Dr Haynes could not feel any pedal pulses. The dorsalis pedis pulse was palpable on the right foot. Dr Haynes admitted Reg urgently to hospital.

In hospital Reg was found to have a popliteal aneurysm with an embolism in the left foot. Thrombolysis was unsuccessful and the patient had a below the knee amputation. He sued Dr Berg and Dr Haynes for an allegedly negligent delay in diagnosis of an acutely ischaemic foot.

 Expert opinion

A painful red foot may be caused by a number of conditions including infection (cellulitis, infective arthritis and osteomyelitis), inflammation (gout and other arthropathies) and ischaemia.

Asymptomatic peripheral arterial disease is very common in older patients. In one US screening study 14% of asymptomatic men and women aged 55 and over who were screened had chronic peripheral arterial disease manifested as reduced pulse pressure in the pedal arteries (McGrae *et al.*, 2001).

General practitioners see chronic incomplete ischaemia quite commonly (Cassar, 2006) but only rarely see the acute or acute on chronic severely or 'completely' ischaemic leg (Humphreys, 1999).

Limb ischaemia is usually classified in terms of the time of its onset and its severity. The classification is reproduced in Case Table 17.1 from Callum and Bradbury (2000).

Generations of medical students have been taught the '6 P's' of the acutely ischaemic foot;

- pain
- pallor
- pulseless
- perishing cold
- paraesthesia
- paralysis.

Paraesthesia and paralysis are discriminatory for complete ischaemia but are rare unless the ischaemia is very severe.

If chronic peripheral arterial disease causes symptoms the patient sometimes complains of a cold or discoloured foot but usually complains of intermittent claudication. Rest pain, occurring in the foot at night when the leg is elevated and relieved by dropping the foot over the side of the bed, signifies critical ischaemia. Presumably the residual arterial pressure overcoming the resistance of narrowed vessels is so low that it is augmented by gravity when the foot is in the dependent position.

On examination the acutely ischaemic foot is classically pale and cold. However, it may also be red, and warm and this can cause errors (Humphreys, 1999).

Avoiding Errors in General Practice, First Edition. Kevin Barraclough, Jenny du Toit, Jeremy Budd, Joseph E. Raine, Kate Williams and Jonathan Bonser.
© 2013 John Wiley & Sons, Ltd. Published 2013 by John Wiley & Sons, Ltd.

Case Table 17.1 Classification of limb ischaemia.

Classification of limb ischaemia	
Terminology	Definition or comment
Onset:	
Acute	Ischaemia < 14 days
Acute on chronic	Worsening symptoms and signs (< 14 days)
Chronic	Ischaemia stable for > 14 days
Severity (acute, acute on chronic):	
Incomplete	Limb not threatened
Complete	Limb threatened
Irreversible	Limb non-viable

The temperature of the limb is not always a reliable sign of the severity of ischaemia because it will depend on the ambient temperature, whether the foot was clothed in a sock and so on. Nevertheless, it is unusual to find asymmetric coolness on palpating a lower limb. Such a finding should put a general practitioner on notice that critical or acute arterial ischaemia needs to be excluded.

Dr Berg 'prematurely anchored' on an incorrect diagnosis that was based on an inadequate history and examination. He should have sought a history of intermittent claudication and rest pain. The patient had risk factors of cardiovascular disease. Dr Berg should have noted signs of chronic ischaemia and examined and recorded:

- the relative temperature of the foot;
- the capillary return time by squeezing the under surface of the big toe for 5 seconds and then releasing the pressure; the time in seconds it takes for the normal skin colour to return is the CRT; more than 5 seconds is abnormal; the test is relatively insensitive (it is absent in many cases of peripheral arterial disease) (McGee, 1998);
- whether the foot became pale on elevation;
- the presence or absence of pedal pulses.

Usually the most useful sign for the general practitioner is the presence or absence of palpable peripheral pulses. The acutely ischaemic foot will, for the purposes of a general practitioner, almost always be pulseless.

However, there are two caveats to this assertion:

1. Some authors point to studies that demonstrate that pulses can be present, even in a critically ischaemic foot (McGee & Boyko, 1998). However, the paper cited for this assertion was in patients with diabetes mellitus who may have microvascular disease causing tissue ischaemia rather than macrovascular disease (Boyko *et al.*, 1997). This is not usually the case in the non diabetic population.

2. Palpation of peripheral pulses is not always easy. It is relatively easy for the examiner to mistake the pulsations in the examiner's finger for the patient's pulse if the patient's pulse is of low volume or absent. Studies indicate that agreement between experienced clinicians on the presence or absence of low volume pulses is not perfect. (McGee & Boyko, 1998).

If there is any doubt a hand held Doppler should be used. With the Doppler it is not only possible to detect the presence or absence of pedal pulses. The Ankle Brachial Pressure Index (ABPI) can be calculated. An APBI of ≤ 0.5 is suggestive of critical ischaemia (Humphreys, 1999).

If the history and examination detailed above had been performed Reg would have been referred for an urgent vascular opinion.

Dr Haynes failed to recognize the significance of the numbness of Reg's foot. She was influenced merely by the colour of the foot. The fact that the urate level was slightly raised would not be reassuring. A urate level can be normal in an acute attack of gout (Underwood, 2006) and most patients with hyperuricaemia do not have gout (*DTB*, 2004). Reg was taking bendroflumethiazide which can cause a raised urate level. Dr Haynes also failed to adequately assess the arterial circulation in Reg's foot.

When Reg was seen on the third occasion it had become more obvious that the foot was ischaemic. The foot did not feel particularly cold because Reg was in bed. However in view of the other clinical findings Dr Haynes rightly admitted him.

 Legal comment

Expert opinion says that Dr Berg was negligent at the first consultation. His examination was inadequate but in particular he failed to check the pedal pulses. If a proper examination had been carried out, we are told that Reg would have been sent urgently to hospital.

As it was, Dr Haynes then negligently lost another opportunity for an urgent referral three days later. So seven days elapsed before Reg was eventually seen urgently. By that time below the knee amputation was required.

The question which will occupy the doctors' MDOs will be, if Reg had been referred promptly, what would the outcome have been on the balance of probability?

They will instruct a vascular expert to report on this question. That expert will be able to review Reg's hospital records, and will have to make an assessment of his probable prognosis seven days before he was actually seen.

If the outcome would probably have been the same, then Reg's claim will be relatively small one for the pain and suffering over the seven days he was not properly treated. If amputation would probably have been avoided, then Reg could expect compensation in the region of £50 000 for pain and suffering, plus the cost of any equipment and care he may need to assist his mobility for the rest of his life.

 Key learning points

Specific to the case

• When assessing a painful red foot always consider ischaemia in the differential diagnosis.

• The most important and sensitive discriminants between critical 'complete' ischaemia and chronic 'incomplete' ischaemia are probably the presence or absence of rest pain and the presence or absence of any (reliably) palpable pedal pulses.

• Access to a handheld Doppler is extremely helpful. (Most GP practices have them so that the practice nurse can perform 4-layer bandaging.)

General point

• Avoid prematurely anchoring on a diagnosis without full assessment and consideration of a differential diagnosis.

References and further reading

Boyko EJ, Ahroni JH, Davignon D, Stensel V, Prigeon RL, Smith DG (1997) Diagnostic utility of the history and physical examination for peripheral vascular disease among patients with diabetes mellitus. *Journal of Clinical Epidemiology* **50**: 659–68.

Callum K, Bradbury A (2000) ABC of arterial and venous disease: Acute limb ischaemia. *BMJ* **320**: 764–7.

Cassar K (2006). Intermittent Claudication. *BMJ* **333**: 1002–5.

DTB (2004) Gout in primary care. *DTP* **42**: 37–40.

Humphreys W (1999) Lesson of the week: The painful red foot-inflammation or ischaemia? *BMJ* **318**: 925–6.

McGee SR, Boyko EJ (1998) Physical examination and chronic lower-extremity ischemia: a critical review. *Arch Intern Med* **158**: 1357–64.

McGrae McDermot M, Kerwin DR, Liu K, Martin GJ, O'Brien E, Kaplan H and Greenland P (2001) Prevalence and significance of unrecognised lower extremity peripheral arterial disease in general medicine practice. *J Gen Inter Med* **16**: 384–90.

Underwood M (2006) Diagnosis and management of gout. *BMJ* **332**: 1315–19.

Case 18 A flare-up of ulcerative colitis

Jenny was diagnosed with ulcerative colitis, localized to the rectum when she was aged 32. She was initially followed up in the gastroenterology clinic but after two years was discharged to her general practitioner. She managed her relatively mild symptoms with intermittent use of mesalazine 1g enemas.

At the age of 37 she gave up smoking and experienced a flare up of her symptoms. She consulted Dr Jones about the problem. Dr Jones noted a two-week history of worsening diarrhoea and abdominal pain. She noted that abdominal examination was normal.

What would you do now?

Dr Jones suggested stopping the mesalazine enemas and using prednisolone retention enemas 20 mg once daily instead. She advised Jenny to return if the symptoms did not settle.

Ten days later Jenny returned. Dr Jones recorded that the symptoms were no better. She started oral mesalazine slow release 400 mg and loperamide 4 mg each three times daily. She told Jenny to return if the symptoms did not settle.

What would be your differential diagnosis and how would you discriminate between them?

One week later Jenny requested a home visit. One of Dr Jones' colleagues visited her at home, noted that she was opening her bowels 12 times daily, had a temperature of 38 °C and was dehydrated with a resting pulse of 112 bpm and a blood pressure of 100/60 mmHg. Jenny was admitted to hospital and two days later underwent a total colectomy for a toxic megacolon.

Jenny brought a claim against Dr Jones alleging that her assessment was inadequate and that a competent general practitioner would have treated her symptoms more aggressively initially and sought urgent specialist opinion if the symptoms failed to settle.

Do you think her claim will succeed?

Expert comment

Delayed diagnosis of toxic megacolon in a patient with ulcerative colitis is a regular allegation in medico-legal cases. It may occur with an initial presentation of ulcerative colitis (Case 8) or occur, and fail to be recognized, in a patient with known ulcerative colitis.

It is relatively common for general practitioners to have to manage conditions that are usually managed in specialist clinics. The patient may have been discharged from specialist care (as in this case) or it may be that the patient cannot contact the specialist clinic or merely seeks advice about the condition closer to home.

Ulcerative colitis affects about 1 in 1000 of the population so most general practitioners will have a few patients with the condition. However, it is an example of a condition that is usually managed in specialist clinics. If a general practitioner decides to intervene and manage the patient it is necessary to be competent to do so. It may be that the general practitioner has quite a lot of experience of the condition or the general practitioner may seek information from the sources such as the BNF, review articles in journals or other authoritative online medical resources.

In this case there were various problems with Dr Jones's management.

There is a well-established system for categorizing the severity of a flare up of ulcerative colitis. This has been outlined in review articles in the *BMJ* (Collins & Rhodes, 2006) and is detailed in online UK resources such as Prodigy and the CKS database. This is outlined in Case Box 18.1.

Case Box 18.1   Disease severity of ulcerative colitis

Mild

Fewer than four stools daily, with or without blood

No systemic disturbance

Normal erythrocyte sedimentation rate and C reactive protein values

Moderate

Four to six stools a day with minimal systemic disturbance

Severe

More than six stools a day containing blood and evidence of systemic disturbance (fever, tachycardia, anaemia, or hypoalbuminaemia)

Dr Jones did note record essential bits of information such as, particularly, stool frequency, the presence or absence of blood in the stool, weight loss or abdominal pain. It was not recorded whether Jenny was well or unwell and what her pulse, temperature and blood pressure was. Dr Jones recalled that Jenny did not seem particularly unwell but there was nothing to corroborate this impression and noting to show that Dr Jones had carried out an adequate assessment.

Guidance suggests measuring inflammatory markers such as ESR and CRP plus indicators of disease severity such as serum albumin. The exacerbation could be due to bacterial gastroenteritis or C Difficile and guidance recommends stool culture are obtained to exclude infection.

There was also evidence that Dr Jones had not read, or was not familiar with, standard treatment of a relapse of ulcerative colitis.

Mesalazine suppositories are considered to be probably more rather than less effective than prednisolone enemas and the guidance indicates that topical agents on their own are unlikely to be effective alone. Guidance articles suggest adding in oral mesalazine in doses of more than 3 g (rather than 1.2 g). The BNF and all guidance advise against the use of loperamide or codeine phosphate in ulcerative colitis as these agents increase the risk of toxic megacolon.

Dr Jones's level of monitoring and follow up ('see if it does not settle') also did not show adequate awareness of the risk of toxic megacolon and the fact that nearly a third of patients with ulcerative colitis end up having to have a total colectomy.

Overall, the evidence was that Dr Jones did not really adequately assess Jenny and did not show competence in the initial management of a flare-up of ulcerative colitis. It would have been reasonable to either seek specialist advice immediately or follow standard guidance about assessment and initial management and seek specialist advice if remission was not induced within one to two weeks.

 Legal comment

A GP is judged according to the standards of an ordinary competent GP. Of course, some GPs may have more expertise than others in managing certain conditions. The important point is to be able to recognize the limits of one's competence. It looks as if Dr Jones exceeded the limits of her expertise, with the result that there has been a breach of duty to Jenny. She is therefore liable to Jenny for all the consequences of that breach, which include the removal of her colon, any associated pain and suffering and (possibly) any psychiatric consequences.

It is difficult to assess the value of this claim without knowing a lot more about the circumstances. Dr Jones's lawyers will no doubt make the point that Jenny's colon was already compromised by her illness. However, Jenny's claim could well be worth tens of thousands of pounds.

 Key learning points

Specific to the case

• Ulcerative colitis is normally treated in specialist clinics. Approximately one third of suffers with a pancolitis end up needing a total colectomy (Carter *et al.*, 2004).

• There are relatively simple guidelines for assessing severity and initiating treatment that a general practitioner should look up or be aware of if he/she is going to initially assess and treat a relapse of mild to moderate severity.

• Antidiarrhoeal agents should not be used.

General points
- General practitioners are often consulted about exacerbations of chronic conditions like ulcerative colitis that are usually managed in specialist clinics.
- It is important to seek immediate specialist advice or to consult up to date guidance and be competent before intervening in any way.

References

Carter MJ, Lobo AJ, Travis SPL (2004) Guidelines for the management of inflammatory bowel disease in adults. *GUT* **53**: 1–16.

Collins P, Rhodes J (2006) Ulcerative colitis: diagnosis and management. *BMJ* **333**: 340–3.

Case 19 A woman with a skin lump on her leg

Martha was 35 years old when she consulted Dr Welch about contraception and also took the opportunity to mention a small lump on one of her calves. She mentioned the possibility of an insect bite on her lower leg which had occasionally been 'weepy' and had occasionally been scratched and bled. Dr Welch recorded '?pyogenic granuloma'. He recommended that Martha attend the practice's Nurse Practitioner-run cryotherapy clinic.

Martha did this a couple of weeks later and the treatment appeared uneventful.

About a year later Martha presented with a lump in the groin. This proved to be due to metastatic amelanotic malignant melanoma, which was also confirmed in a small nodule at the site of the original cryotherapy. Unfortunately the disease was not treatable.

Before she died, Martha commenced a claim against Dr Welch.

Do you think a claim against Dr Welch will succeed?

 Expert comment

Pyogenic granulomas are not common skin lesions. They tend to occur on the hand, lips, face or shoulder region. They are unusual on the lower leg.

Cryotherapy is a popular method of treating warts and other benign skin lesions. The difference, however, between cryotherapy and many other methods of treating skin lesions is that no tissue is available for histology. Therefore the diagnosis must be known with a high degree of certainty (which often is the case with skin tags, seborrhoeic keratoses and viral warts).

A pyogenic granuloma should not be treated with cryotherapy because, without histological confirmation, it may be an amelanotic malignant melanoma.

NICE guidelines suggest the use of a 7-point checklist with suspected malignant melanomas: looking for change in size, irregular shape, irregular colour, largest diameter 7 mm or more, inflammation, oozing, change in sensation. One problem is that the sensitivity of this clinical prediction rule is very low (around 40–50%) (Abbasi *et al.*, 2004). A significant proportion of the pigmented lesions a general practitioner examines routinely should be referred urgently if the rule is strictly adhered to.

However, in this case the lesion was not pigmented. It was also on the lower leg in a woman. This is quite a common place for a malignant melanoma in women (the shoulders are commoner places for men). However, Dr Welch may quite reasonably not have even thought of the possibility that the nonpigmented lesion could be a malignant melanoma. Amelanotic melanomas are rare, and they are often described as 'the great masquerader' in skin lesions (Koch & Lange, 2000). Nevertheless, amelanotic melanomas are frequently misdiagnosed as pyogenic granulomas.

There are several potential criticisms of Dr Welch's management which exemplify some of the types of cognitive error that may occur.

A probable source of error in this case was 'premature anchoring' bias – the tendency to begin from the assumption that a nonpigmented nodular skin lesion could not be a malignant melanoma. This form of cognitive error can be compounded by 'confirmation bias': the tendency to look for information that would be consistent with the preferred diagnosis, rather than information which would refute it. The lesion looks like the pictures of pyogenic granulomas in dermatology texts.

However, in this case the lesion was single, and it was on the calf. The site was therefore less usual for a pyogenic granuloma. A pyogenic granuloma has a differential diagnosis associated with it which includes amelanotic melanoma. It was necessary to 'second guess' the presumed diagnosis. Also, the information that the lesion had occasionally been weepy and bled was ignored.

Avoiding Errors in General Practice, First Edition. Kevin Barraclough, Jenny du Toit, Jeremy Budd, Joseph E. Raine, Kate Williams and Jonathan Bonser.
© 2013 John Wiley & Sons, Ltd. Published 2013 by John Wiley & Sons, Ltd.

Dr Welch had not recorded any history (duration, change in size or appearance) which would suggest that he had considered alternative diagnoses.

Realistically, it was a mistake to deal with the lesion by cryotherapy: any treatment method that gave tissue for histology would have been acceptable.

 ## Legal comment

When the GP expert looks at Dr Welch's very brief note ('?pyogenic granuloma') that will probably be enough for him to recommend that the case will be indefensible on breach of duty. Even if Dr Welch were to recall a number of reassuring circumstances to justify his decision to treat with cryotherapy, the fact he did not record them makes his position very weak indeed.

By contrast, Martha's lawyers will take a detailed witness statement from her before she dies. It will describe the history of the lump and the consultation with Dr Welch. If she dies before the trial, that witness statement will stand as her evidence, even though it cannot be cross examined.

A dermatologist may conclude that earlier treatment of the melanoma would not have saved Martha's life. But there was a delay of a year before she received treatment and so it seems likely that such an expert will conclude that earlier treatment would have made a difference.

The circumstances are overwhelmingly against Dr Welch. His MDO will want to settle the case on the best possible terms. If Martha is married and has children who are now deprived of a mother the case will be potentially expensive: well over £100 000. If not, then its

value is limited to compensation for her suffering before death and the cost of care that she will have needed as her condition deteriorated.

 ## Key learning points

Specific to the case
• When diagnosing rare skin lesions it is necessary to be very careful that one is aware of the standard differential diagnoses.
• Lesions with uncertain differentials, such as presumed pyogenic granulomas, need to be fully excised and sent for histological diagnosis.

General points
• Always 'second guess' and consider the differential diagnoses.

References and further reading

Abbasi NR, Shaw HM, Rigel DS, Friedman RJ, McCarthy WH, Osman I, *et al.* (2004) Early diagnosis of cutaneous melanoma: revisiting the ABCD criteria. *JAMA* **292**: 2771–6.

Andrews MD (2004) Cryosurgery for common skin conditions. *Am Fam Physician* **69**(10): 2365–72.

Koch SE, Lange JR (2000) Amelanotic melanoma: The great masquerader. *Journal of the American Academy of Dermatology* **42**: 731–4.

NICE (2005) Guideline CG027 on the recognition of malignant melanoma.

Case 20 A woman with microscopic haematuria

Alice was 56 when she consulted Dr Hendry. She had been feeling nonspecifically unwell with fatigue, poor sleep and headaches. In the course of examining her Dr Hendry found Alice's blood pressure was 176/100 mmHg. Dr Hendry arranged for Alice to see the practice nurse for three blood pressure checks, blood tests and ECG and urinalysis. Alice's blood pressure was satisfactory, her blood tests and ECG were normal and urinalysis showed 2 + blood. The practice nurse sent the urine sample off for microscopy and culture and this showed no growth and no cells.

What would you do now?

Alice consulted another partner a few months later. She had malaise and dysuria. Urinalysis showed blood, protein and leucocytes and she was treated for a urine infection. No follow up urine sample was sent. This pattern was repeated a year later.

At the age of 58 Alice underwent an insurance medical and was noted to have 3 + microscopic haematuria.

What would be your differential diagnosis and how would you discriminate between them?

The insurance report was sent to the practice but no action was taken. On her 59th birthday Alice was admitted into hospital with fever, vomiting and left renal colic. She was found to have a left hydronephrosis secondary to a stage 3 bladder cancer.

Alice brought a claim against Dr Hendry and the practice for failure to investigate persistent microscopic haematuria.

Do you think her claim will succeed?

 ### Expert comment

Microscopic haematuria is a difficult condition for general practitioners because it is very common but can indicate serious disease. In the UK the July 2000 Referral Guidelines for Suspected Cancer (the 'Two Week Rule' referrals) recommended urgent referral of all patients with microscopic haematuria over the age of 50. In the June 2005 version this was changed to 'unexplained' microscopic haematuria.

The difficulty with this is that microscopic haematuria is relatively common and until recently it has been rather poorly defined. A 2003 review in the *New England Journal of Medicine* found studies quoting prevalence rates that varied from 0.18% to 16.1% (Cohen & Brown, 2003). Older studies suggest that 4% to 7% of the general population will have microscopic haematuria. One 1986 US study found a prevalence of 13% in asymptomatic males and females over the age of 50. On investigation 2.3% of those investigated had serious disease and 0.5% had renal or bladder cancer (Mohr et al., 1986).

More recent guidance has advised that the terms non visible and visible haematuria replace the terms microscopic and macroscopic. Nonvisible haematuria includes dipstick haematuria of more than a trace of blood and red cells detected on urine microscopy. Urinalysis (of 1 + or more) appears to detect levels of haematuria equivalent to 3–5 red cells per high-powered microscopy field (roughly the previous definition of haematuria). It is not necessary to confirm with urine microscopy (Kelly et al., 2009).

Common causes of nonvisible haematuria are menstruation, sexual intercourse and urinary tract infection (UTI). These need to be excluded before any other investigation. Athletes such as long-distance runners get nonvisible haematuria and should probably be reinvestigated after three days' abstention from activities.

Avoiding Errors in General Practice, First Edition. Kevin Barraclough, Jenny du Toit, Jeremy Budd, Joseph E. Raine, Kate Williams and Jonathan Bonser.
© 2013 John Wiley & Sons, Ltd. Published 2013 by John Wiley & Sons, Ltd.

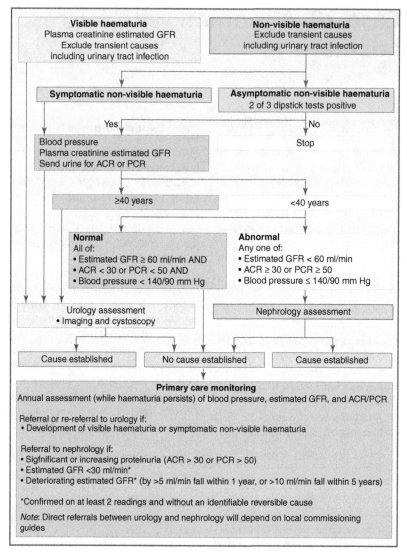

Case Figure 20.1 Assessment and management of non-visible haematuria in primary care.
Source: Kelly KD, Fawcett DP, Goldberg LC (2009) Assessment and management of non-visible haematuria in primary care. *BMJ* **388**: bmj.a3021.

Persistent unexplained nonvisible haematuria can be caused by glomerular renal disease (most often IgA nephropathy or thin basement membrane disease) or urological disease such as stones or cancer.

Recent guidance is that nonvisible haematuria in asymptomatic patients should be confirmed on two out of three urinalysis tests before being investigated. After treatment of a UTI with nonvisible haematuria urinalysis should be repeated and investigated if the haematuria is persistent. A 2009 algorithm by Kelly *et al.* (2009) is reproduced in Case Figure 20.1:

In this case it is clear that Alice had persistent microscopic haematuria that was not investigated. Dr Hendry was reassured on the first occasion that urine microscopy did not pick up any red cells. However, haematuria is often intermittent and the urinalysis was likely to be correct. It should really have been repeated at twice. The second and third episodes occurred within the context of UTIs but UTIs may be secondary to underlying urological disease and the general practitioners should really have checked that the haematuria cleared after treatment. On the last occasion the information from the insurance report should really have been acted upon.

Legal comment

Expert opinion suggests it will be hard to defend the practice for its failure to respond to the findings of the insurance medical. This is even though it seems that Alice did not come to the practice to ask for advice. The expert implies that a positive duty lay on the practice to contact Alice in the light of that report, particularly given her history.

Expert opinion also suggests there may have been breaches of duty by the GPs on previous occasions over the last two years or so, when further analysis should have been done, which might have highlighted under-lying urological disease.

However, the expert might be asked by the lawyers acting for the GPs (and their MDOs) to express a view on whether there is a responsible body of GP opinion which might have acted as the GPs in this saga did. After all, it might be pointed out, microscopic haematuria is very common. Is it realistic, given resources, to follow all such patients up? Published guidance is all very well, it might be argued, but does it not represent an ideal rather than a basic required standard?

These are the kinds of discussions which will take place at meetings with Dr Hendry and her partner(s), before it is decided whether to concede or resist this claim. Generally, though, expert opinion in support of the doctors will need to be robust if the MDO is to defend the claim. That looks rather unlikely in this case.

Key learning points

Specific to the case

• Asymptomatic 'microscopic haematuria' is a common and rather difficult finding in primary care. In the past it has suffered from nonuniform definitions of and large variations in published prevalence rates and predictive values for disease.

• Before investigation spurious causes such as menstruation, sexual intercourse and UTI should be excluded and it should be confirmed as being present in two out of three samples. Urinalysis haematuria of 1 + or more has the same significance as the finding on urine microscopy.

• More recent guidance advises the use of the term 'nonvisible haematuria' and advises an investigation algorithm reproduced above.

• Persistent unexplained nonvisible haematuria (two out of three samples) in someone over the age of 50 requires urgent referral under the NICE 2005 guidance.

• Nonvisible haematuria within the context of a UTI should really be rechecked after treatment to check that it has cleared.

General points

• Minor unexpected abnormalities on testing are relatively common and it is important to have a clear idea in advance which need repeating (such as urinalysis haematuria) and which probably do not (such as a serum sodium of 132 mmol/l).

• It is relatively common in medico-legal cases to see abnormal results from private screening facilities (the 'BUPA check') or insurance medicals that the practice is notified about but fails to act upon.

References

Cohen R, Brown R (2003) Microscopic hematuria. *N Engl J Med* **348**: 2330–8.

Kelly KD, Fawcett DP, Goldberg LC (2009) Assessment and management of non-visible haematuria in primary care. *BMJ* **388**: bmj.a3021.

Mohr DN, Offord KP, Owen RA, Melton LJ (1986) Asymptomatic microhematuria and urologic disease. *JAMA: The Journal of the American Medical Association* **256**: 224–9.

Case 21 A limping young girl

Anna was born by full-term normal vaginal delivery. Her Apgar scores were fine and she was discharged three days after delivery, having been examined by the paediatric SHO. Dr Callard carried out her 6-week check, and noted her hips were normal. Her 9-month check was also normal.

At 15 months Anna's mother brought her to see Dr James because she seemed to have difficulty walking. Her mother thought that she walked on the outside of her foot. Dr James examined Anna and could not detect any abnormality. He suggested that it was probably because Anna had only recently started walking and advised mother to see how things progressed and to bring Anna back if there were problems.

What would you do now?

Twelve months later one of Anna's mother's friends, who was a health visitor, suggested Anna was reviewed. Dr James referred her for physiotherapy. The physiotherapist noted that Anna limped, that the right leg was shorter than the left and that there was a restricted range of movement at the right hip. She was referred for an orthopaedic opinion and X-ray demonstrated a right dislocated hip. A month later Anna underwent an open reduction of the right hip, Salter osteotomy and was placed in a Spica cast.

Anna's mother brought a claim against the hospital, the practice, Dr Callard and Dr James alleging that Anna's Developmental Disorder of the Hip (DDH) should have picked up by the screening procedure and by Dr James' examination when Anna was aged 15 months.

Do you think her claim will succeed?

 Expert comment

Cases of delayed diagnosis of Developmental Disorder of the Hip (DDH) are relatively common causes of claims against general practitioners.

Since 1969 there has been a program in the UK for screening babies for Congenital Dislocation of the Hip (CDH).

At birth and six weeks the examiner carries out the Barlow and Ortolani manoeuvres. These tests aim to dislocate an unstable hip and relocate a dislocated hip respectively. By three months these tests do not work (due to contractures in the hip musculature).

It is estimated that only 35% of cases of CDH or DDH are detected by this clinical screening method without ultrasound (Dezateux et al., 2003). However, the concern is that universal ultrasound screening may lead to over diagnosis and treatment of children who would be better untreated. Consequently, routine ultrasound examination of the hips is only carried out in children with risk factors for DDH (a family history of the condition, infants presenting by the breech, other congenital postural deformities, such as those of the foot, oligohydramnios, a history of intrauterine fetal growth retardation).

In the unscreened population many cases of DDH will not be detected at birth or at the 6–8 week check.

In these children the condition may be noticed before the child is walking, because of asymmetry of skin creases at the buttocks and top of the thigh. The condition may also be suspected if the child is limping once he/she starts walking. At that stage clinical examination may demonstrate asymmetric skin folds, leg length shortening on the affected side and a reduced range of movement (particularly abduction) on the affected side.

If a general practitioner suspects DDH in a child in the first three months of life then urgent specialist referral is required because there is good evidence that delay in treatment affects outcome.

By the time the child is aged over 1 there is less urgency required in seeking specialist opinion but any general practitioner does need to have a high index of suspicion for DDH (as screening misses many cases). If the condition is suspected (with, for example, a limping

Avoiding Errors in General Practice, First Edition. Kevin Barraclough, Jenny du Toit, Jeremy Budd, Joseph E. Raine, Kate Williams and Jonathan Bonser.
© 2013 John Wiley & Sons, Ltd. Published 2013 by John Wiley & Sons, Ltd.

child) the general practitioner must examine the child carefully, looking in particular for an abnormal gait, asymmetric skin creases, leg length difference but most importantly the symmetry and range of hip abduction.

If the examination is abnormal then a competent general practitioner would refer for a specialist orthopaedic opinion and may refer for an X-ray of the hip. If the examination is completely normal then a general practitioner should really arrange review in a few weeks to make sure that any gait abnormality has completely resolved and refer if it has not.

In this case it would be difficult to sustain criticism of the hospital, the 6-week check or the 9-month check. The sensitivity of the screening examinations is too low to conclude that, because the condition was missed, the examination was not carried out competently. Even in competent hands only 35% will be detected with clinical screening without ultrasound.

However, once a 13-month-old child is perceived to have an abnormal gait by her mother it is clearly necessary to consider the possibility of DDH since an abnormal gait when a child starts walking is a common presentation of DDH in those in whom screening has missed the condition.

It is necessary to examine the child's gait, observe for skin crease symmetry, check for leg length differences and, most importantly, check that hip abduction is symmetric.

A difficulty in this case was that Dr James's clinical notes were brief and merely recorded 'O/E NAD'. An orthopaedic expert concluded that, when Dr James saw her at 15 months, Anna would have had a shortened right leg, asymmetric thigh and buttock skin creases and reduced right hip abduction. These clinical features should have been apparent in a competent examination by a general practitioner and so Dr James was considered in breach of duty.

The Claimant may have difficulty proving significant harm flowed from this breach of duty because DDH diagnosed at 15 months would still require operative reduction. The main causation case was dependent on proving breach of duty in the first 3 months, which was not done.

 Legal comment

The expert opinion is that Dr James's examination when Anna was 15 months old must have been negligent,

because there would have been obvious signs of DDH. The excessively brief note made by him tends to confirm an impression of a cursory examination.

However, as surgery was inevitable anyway by that time, it seems that the only harm done is that Anna may have been uncomfortable for longer than necessary.

So Anna's mother should be advised that any damages payable are of a relatively small order. Her lawyers should encourage her to settle the case for a modest sum.

 Key learning points

Specific to the case
- Delayed diagnosis of DDH is a common cause of negligence actions against general practitioners.
- It is necessary to be aware that standard clinical screening, carried out competently, will miss a third of cases.
- Because of this it is necessary to assess any report of asymmetry of legs or any abnormality of gait in a young child very carefully. The key signs to look for are asymmetric thigh or buttock creases, objective evidence of thigh to knee length difference (the Galeazzi test) and, most crucially limitation of hip abduction.
- The signs are particularly difficult if the dislocation is bilateral.

General points
- The diagnostic error often occurs because the condition has not been seen before by the general practitioner.

References and further reading

Dezateux C, Brown J, Arthur R, Karnon J, Parnaby A (2003) Performance, treatment pathways, and effects of alternative policy options for screening for developmental dysplasia of the hip in the United Kingdom. *Arch Dis Child* **88**: 753–9.

Sewell MD, Rosendahl K, Eastwood DM (2009) Developmental dysplasia of the hip. *BMJ* **339**: b4454.

Case 22 A builder tripping over his feet

Tom was a 58-year-old man who ran his own business as a builder. He visited Dr Tugwell complaining that his legs felt heavy. There was no pain. He had previously had osteoarthrosis symptoms in the knees and left hip, and occasionally had low back pain. He had had mild left-sided hand symptoms on and off, suggestive of carpal tunnel syndrome. Dr Tugwell recorded that foot pulses were normal and the legs were 'neuro nad'. No specific diagnosis was made.

Three months later Tom came back and said that his legs still felt heavy and that it was beginning to trouble him at work. He seemed to trip a lot and was finding ladders difficult. Dr Tugwell examined his knees and hip joints and thought the symptoms were probably a manifestation of arthritis. Naproxen was prescribed.

What would be your differential diagnosis and how would you discriminate between them?

Tom attended A&E a few weeks later. He had accidentally lost his grip on a heavy bucket of cement and dropped it on his foot. When seeing Dr Tugwell for a medical certificate a week later, he commented that he must be getting old because he had never had an accident of the sort before. He commented on his difficulty in walking and Dr Tugwell agreed that this was probably due to the injury to his foot.

Two weeks later Tom consulted the practice registrar, Dr Phillips. He reported increased difficulty passing urine over some months, but a particular difficulty in the last week or so. Dr Phillips did a digital rectal examination and diagnosed benign prostatic hypertrophy. He arranged for a deferred PSA and started him on an alpha blocker.

Tom next consulted Dr Atwell two months later. He was noticing a continuing tendency to drop things. He felt his grip was weak. Dr Atwell examined his hands and could find no specific abnormality but agreed to make a referral for nerve conduction studies. Dr Atwell noticed the Tom's gait appeared awkward but did not examine him since Tom thought it was due to his foot injury. He requested another X-ray of the foot to exclude a fracture. This was normal.

When Tom attended several weeks later for the nerve conduction studies, the neurophysiologist was so concerned by the patient's gait that he asked a neurology registrar to see the patient. The registrar noted that Tom had urinary symptoms and that for some months he had had electric shock symptoms in his legs if he bent his neck. He found that power was largely normal but there was symmetrically increased tone in the legs with very brisk knee and ankle reflexes, sustained bilateral ankle and knee clonus and upgoing plantar reflexes. There were no objective sensory signs.

An urgent MRI scan revealed a compressive myelopathy in the cervical spine secondary to a spondyltic bar at the C4/5 level. Decompression surgery was carried out soon after but Tom made only marginal improvement and he had to give up his business.

Tom instructed solicitors who were critical of the failure to record a neurological examination of the legs over a period of some 8 months between the first consultation and the eventual diagnosis.

Do you think his claim will succeed?

 Expert comment

Cervical spondylosis is very common in the older population and can present in one of three ways:
1. axial neck pain with restricted rotation (extremely common);
2. cervical radiculopathy (compression of the cervical nerve root); this is not uncommon;

Avoiding Errors in General Practice, First Edition. Kevin Barraclough, Jenny du Toit, Jeremy Budd, Joseph E. Raine, Kate Williams and Jonathan Bonser.

3. compression of the spinal cord itself (cervical myelopathy) which is rare except in the very elderly.

Cervical myelopathy is uncommonly seen in general practice. It tends to present insidiously. It gets commoner with age, since the cause is usually degenerative disease in the cervical spine. Occasionally, though, the cervical myelopathy presents in younger patients with soft prolapsed cervical discs (Bentley *et al.*, 2001). The presentation may begin with either upper limb or lower limb symptoms although eventually both are involved. Nonspecific complaints of leg heaviness or weakness are common, as is unsteady gait, and clumsy or weak hands. Neck stiffness is also common but is not (as here) necessarily a complaint.

Another symptom is 'Lhermitte's sign'. It is sometimes called the 'barber shop sign'. It was originally described in the 1920s in patients with multiple sclerosis affecting the brainstem or cervical cord. The term refers to the symptoms of showers of electric shock type symptoms passing down the torso into the legs on flexion of the neck.

Gait symptoms, trips and falls, and clumsiness in the hands often precede obvious signs by months or years. Objective signs, when they occur, are of lower motor neurone signs in the arms and upper motor neurone signs in the legs. Rarely, there may be a sensory level on the torso.

In this case the three general practitioners (and the A&E doctor) were at fault because no examination of the patient's legs had been made over a period of some 8 months. It was naturally uncertain at what time there would have been signs (increased reflexes, upgoing plantars, ankle clonus) that a GP would have detected, but examination after the A&E attendance and more probably when the patient was complaining of clumsiness of the hands, may have demonstrated those abnormalities.

General practitioners are often not confident in eliciting neurological signs and not infrequently fail to try. In order to detect a signs such as increased tone in the legs it is necessary to examine a lot of 'normals'. However, a mild spastic paraparesis is particularly difficult because bilaterally brisk reflexes are usually due to the patient being nervous and, in most conditions, it is the asymmetry between right and left that alerts the general practitioner to the abnormality. In addition the older patient often has difficulty relaxing making assessment of tone in the legs difficult. (A tip: if, with the patient on the couch, flicking the knee up causes the ankle to come off the couch – the tone is probably increased. Sustained ankle clonus, and indeed knee clonus, are useful signs if present as they are always abnormal.)

Cervical myelopathy is one of those occasional but serious diagnoses that are much easier to recognize if they are borne in mind: what is sometimes referred to as a 'cognitive forcing strategy'. This is much the same as the checking for 'red flags' that is now second nature to many GPs in dealing with low back pain and sciatica.

In this case the outcome was not too bad. Often the patient slips and gets a minor flexion extension injury to an already compressed cord, the cord is contused and the patient irreversibly paraplegic.

 ## Legal comment

The expert is clear that there has been a breach of duty by both the GP and the doctor in A&E. The next question is what would the outcome have probably been if the cervical myelopathy had been diagnosed sooner?

This is a potentially expensive claim for the GPs. After all, Tom has had to give up his business. Was this the consequence of the breach of duty? If so, there will have to be an analysis of the likely income from his business for the rest of Tom's working life. If Tom has not also sued the hospital, the MDOs of the Defendant GPs will consider whether to seek a contribution from the hospital.

 ## Key learning points

Specific to the case

• General practitioners often find it difficult to assess tone and reflexes, especially in the elderly who find it difficult to relax. It is easier when there is an asymmetry than with a symmetrical spastic paraparesis.

• Sustained ankle clonus and knee clonus are always abnormal signs if elicited.

• With the patient on the couch and flicking the knee up causes the ankle to come off the couch – the tone is probably increased.

• In the patient with a cervical spondylitic myelopathy symptoms may occur quite a lot earlier than signs. Urinary symptoms in someone tripping over pavestones is a clue.

General points

- A cervical myelopathy is one of those diagnoses that are usually missed because the doctor merely failed to think of it.
- 'Cognitive forcing strategies' – making yourself second guess can help to avoid making rare but catastrophic mistakes.

References and further reading

Bentley PI, Grigor CJ, McNally JD, Rigby S, Higgens CS, Frank AO, *et al.* Lesson of the week: Degenerative cervical disc disease causing cord compression in adults under 50. *BMJ* **322**: 414–415.

Patten J (1996) *Neurological Differential Diagnosis*, 2nd Edition, Springer Verlag, Chapter 15.

Case 23 An anxious young woman with hyperventilation

Kathy, about 13 weeks pregnant, consulted Dr Shah complaining of tiredness, recent work stress, and anxiety. She had had cystitis several days previously and been given some antibiotics for that by an Out of Hours service. During the consultation with Dr Shah she appeared anxious and was hyperventilating.

What would you do now?

Dr Shah asked about the onset of her problems, which the patient thought were recent. Dr Shah reviewed the history but there were no previous instances of significant anxiety. There was a discussion about the work problems and Dr Shah advised Kathy to return if the situation did not improve, when blood tests for thyroid function would be considered.

What would be your differential diagnosis and how would you discriminate between them?

Next day Kathy was admitted as an emergency via Accident and Emergency, having collapsed at work. The admitting doctor noted a history of becoming significantly unwell over a couple of weeks with thirst, polyuria and weight loss. In the past few days she had been anxious and breathless. She was diagnosed with diabetic ketoacidosis and was very seriously unwell. However she did recover and required continuing treatment with insulin. Unfortunately the illness caused her to miscarry.

Kathy brought a case against Dr Shah alleging that he should have carried out urinalysis and that this would have avoided her miscarriage.

Do you think her claim will succeed?

 Expert comment

Fortunately the patient survived, but 3–5% of patients with diabetic ketoacidosis (DKA) do still die.

Delayed diagnosis of DKA is a relatively common cause of claims against general practitioners, although the general practitioner may only encounter an undiagnosed diabetic presenting with DKA once or twice in a career.

More commonly the patient is known to have Type 1 diabetes, has been unwell for a few days, and the general practitioner fails to check a urinalysis. This is a commoner but less understandable error. 14% of patients with Type 1 diabetes who are unwell and have a blood glucose over 14 mmol/l will have DKA (Schwab, 1999). If the patient has 1 + ketones or less they can usually be managed in the community with close supervision and advice about 'sick day' insulin rules. If they have 2 + or more ketonuria they need admission. DKA can occur with a blood glucose as low as 14 mmol/l.

What went wrong in this case?

Hyperventilation is a well-recognized component of anxiety. It is associated with 'panic attacks' which may either be reported to the GP or else actually witnessed, often as a result as an urgent request for attention.

However, significant, objectively measured and sustained hyperventilation is not particularly common in primary care (it is probably seen more often in A + E). It is necessary to consider the differential diagnosis.

The differential diagnosis of hyperventilation (i.e. an increase in both respiratory rate and tidal volume) does include anxiety, but also respiratory infections, pulmonary oedema, fever generally, pulmonary embolus, thyrotoxicosis and any cause of metabolic acidosis. Metabolic acidosis in turn can result from sepsis, uraemia, or diabetes.

A person with anxiety who is hyperventilating will commonly (although not always) develop symptoms such as tingling in the hands and feet, and dizziness. There will usually be a prior history of anxiety and panic episodes. The complaint of breathing difficulty will often form part of the presenting complaint, rather than

Avoiding Errors in General Practice, First Edition. Kevin Barraclough, Jenny du Toit, Jeremy Budd, Joseph E. Raine, Kate Williams and Jonathan Bonser.
© 2013 John Wiley & Sons, Ltd. Published 2013 by John Wiley & Sons, Ltd.

(as here) being noticed by the doctor. Patients with anxiety causing hyperventilation are usually seen as an 'urgent' appointment. This patient had made the appointment two days previously. Patients with anxiety-induced hyperventilation usually settle during the course of a medical consultation.

In this case Kathy presented, as many patients do to GPs, with symptoms of tiredness and work stress. Dr Shah assumed that the hyperventilation was the result of this, but did not pay attention to the incongruous features, which were:

- no previous history of anxiety;
- hyperventilation not complained of;
- appointment made 2 days earlier.

It was possible that Kathy's symptoms were hyperventilation due to anxiety. However, Dr Shah needed to consider other possibilities such as pulmonary embolism (she was pregnant), sepsis, thyrotoxicosis or DKA. It was necessary to measure respiratory rate, temperature, pulse and blood pressure. It was necessary to listen to the chest and lungs, check the legs for swelling and carry out urinalysis. Many general practitioners now would check pulse oximetry. Hyperventilation due to anxiety should really be a diagnosis of exclusion.

 Legal comment

It seems that Dr Shah's failure to consider other possible causes of Kathy's hyperventilation has exposed him to this claim for the distress of a miscarriage.

In order to assess the value of the claim, Dr Shah's lawyers will ask Kathy to be examined by a psychiatrist. The case will be settled by reference to evidence of the effect on Kathy of her experience. The compensation could range from about £3000 for minor post-traumatic distress, up to about £12 000 for moderate PTSD, or even more for a severe case.

 Key learning points

Specific to the case
- Hyperventilation due to anxiety should really be a diagnosis of exclusion. Many serious conditions such as pulmonary emboli, pulmonary oedema, pneumonia, thyroxicosis and DKA can present in this way.
- Always check for ketonuria in any sick patient with known Type 1 diabetes.

General points
- Always 'second guess': 'Are there any possibilities I have missed, anything I cannot afford to miss?'

Further reading and references

Diabetic ketoacidosis – http://www.patient.co.uk/doctor/Diabetic-Ketoacidosis.htm

Schwab T, Hendey GW, Soliz TC (1999) Screening for ketonemia in patients with diabetes. *Annals of Emergency Medicine* **34**: 342–6.

Case 24 A slightly raised AST in an Asian woman

Mrs Choudhury was 42 and overweight when she consulted Dr Sastry with multiple symptoms. She had been in the UK for two years, had three children and was very tired, suffered from headaches, nausea, weight gain, abdominal pain, loose stools, palpitations, dizziness and pains in the legs. Dr Sastry considered that, because of her multiple symptoms, Mrs Choudhury could be depressed. However, he decided to check some blood tests including TSH. These showed that Mrs Choudhury had a mild microcytic anaemia which proved to be due to beta thalassaemia trait. Dr Sastry arranged to check her husband. She also had a minimally elevated bilirubin and an AST of 82 IU/L (normal range less than 40).

What would you do now?

Over the next 18 months Mrs Choudhury saw Dr Sastry on many occasions. She suffered from allergic rhinitis, mouth ulcers, head colds, generalized itch, vaginal discomfort, epigastric pain and irregular periods. Upper abdominal ultrasound showed gallstones and a fatty liver. Dr Sastry referred her for a surgical opinion. A repeat ALT 14 months after the original one showed an AST of 90 with a normal bilirubin, albumin and alkaline phosphate.

What would be your differential diagnosis and how would you discriminate between them?

Mrs Choudhury had a laparascopic cholecystectomy but continued to suffer from multiple symptoms. Eventually three years later she began to lose weight, an abdominal ultrasound showed ascites, hepatitis C serology was positive and she was diagnosed with cirrhosis secondary to hepatitis C.

It was alleged that Dr Sastry was negligent in failing to follow up the abnormal liver function tests.

Do you think her claim will succeed?

 Expert comment

The unexpected mildly abnormal blood test result is a very common problem in general practice. Statistically, if the 'normal range' of a test is defined as the mean $+/-$ two standard deviations for the 'normal population' then 5% of the healthy population will fall outside the normal range and if there are 12 results (for example in biochemistry) there is nearly a 50% chance of at least one falling outside the 'normal range' $(1 - 0.95^{12})$. A further difficulty is what Deyo refers to as the 'cascade effects of medical technology' (Deyo, 2002) – the unexpectedly abnormal result leads to further (often unnecessary) investigations and significant patient and clinician anxiety. It is the basis of the old medical adage: 'What is the definition of a normal patient? Someone who has not had enough tests.'

However, in the case of minor abnormalities of liver function tests, which are often ignored, there is an increasing awareness of several causes of chronic hepatitis that are probably increasing in incidence and do have an associated significant morbidity that is potentially avoidable with treatment. These are chronic hepatitis C and B, alcoholic and nonalcoholic steatosis, haemochromatosis and autoimmune hepatitis.

In a Nottingham study Ryder investigated 157 patients who had had LFT requests from primary care in which transaminases or alkaline phosphatase results were more than twice the upper limit of the normal range, had not normalized and were not under investigation. The study investigated these patients and found that 97 (62%) had conditions requiring intervention. The majority had alcoholic liver disease or nonhepatic steatosis but 20 had one of the other conditions listed above (Sherwood et al., 2001). Ryder's recommendation was that, for raised transaminases that are below three

---

Avoiding Errors in General Practice, First Edition. Kevin Barraclough, Jenny du Toit, Jeremy Budd, Joseph E. Raine, Kate Williams and Jonathan Bonser.
© 2013 John Wiley & Sons, Ltd. Published 2013 by John Wiley & Sons, Ltd.

times the upper of limit of normal the test should be repeated in 1 to 3 months and investigated if still raised. The standard initial investigations would be an FBC, ferritin, autoimmune antibodies and hepatitis B and C serology.

As a woman from the Asian subcontinent Mrs Choudhury was at significantly increased risk of chronic hepatitis C. She did have a potential cause for her raised AST results over some years because she was overweight, had a fatty liver and potentially had biliary disease (though the stones may have been asymptomatic). A particular difficulty was also that she was polysymptomatic.

However, a difficulty in this case was that Dr Choudhury had not recorded any reasoning in his interpretation of the raised AST results.

 Legal comment

Dr Sastry and his lawyers will have to analyze this obviously complex case very carefully. It is so easy in hindsight to point to the mistake, but one cannot help but feel rather sorry for him, faced as he was with such an array of symptoms.

After Dr Sastry's solicitor has obtained expert opinion, a meeting will probably be arranged with a barrister and the experts where Dr Sastry will be closely questioned. The lawyers will take into account how well they think he will cope with cross-examination if the case goes to trial.

An expert hepatologist will have to consider whether earlier intervention would have made a difference. It could be that the outcome would not have been significantly altered. If Dr Sastry's expert comes to this conclusion, then whatever his shortcomings, the case could be defended on this causation point alone.

This is a case where there are strengths and weaknesses to the defence. A pragmatic decision will have to be made on whether it will be taken to trial.

 Key learning points

Specific to the case
- Abnormal transaminases or alkaline phosphate are often related to alcohol, non hepatic steatosis or may be related to drugs such as statins. However, when investigated a significant proportion of patients with persistently abnormal results have an underlying liver disorder.
- The conditions to be aware of are chronic hepatitis C and B, alcoholic and nonalcoholic steatosis, haemochromatosis and autoimmune hepatitis.
- There is authoritative guidance that suggests retesting in 1–3 months and investigating if the result is still abnormal.
- The investigations required are FBC, ferritin, autoimmune antibodies and hepatitis serology.

General points
- It is not always easy to deal with the unexpectedly abnormal blood result. It is necessary to avoid over investigation as well as under investigation.
- It is usually good practice to recheck the result at an appropriate interval. The statistical phenomenon of 'regression to the mean' ensures that random variation will usually normalize and persistently abnormal results are not a statistical fluke.

References and further reading

Deyo RA (2002) Cascade effects of medical technology. *Annual Review of Public Health* **23**: 23–44.

Sherwood P, Lyburn I, Brown S, Ryder S (2001) How are abnormal results for liver function tests dealt with in primary care? Audit of yield and impact. *BMJ* **322**: 276–8.

Smellie S, Ryder S (2006) Biochemical 'liver function tests', *BMJ* **333**: 481–3.

Case 25 Cough and fever in a 42-year-old accountant

David was a 42-year-old accountant who kept very fit. His past medical history was unremarkable. He developed an irritating cough and went to see his GP because he was due to go away on holiday. Dr Hope diagnosed an upper respiratory tract infection.

Two days later David contacted the Out of Hours service. He felt feverish, had a headache and was vomiting. He was visited by Dr Jumali who noted that David had felt unwell for a few days, was now generally achy, had vomited and had a headache. He recorded a temperature of 37.1 °C, a pulse of 80, a blood pressure of 140/70, no neck stiffness, and that ENT and respiratory system examinations were normal. Dr Jumali diagnosed a viral illness and advised David to keep his fluid intake up and take regular paracetamol.

Would you have done anything else?

The following afternoon David's wife telephoned the Out of Hours service again. She was concerned that David had been unable to get out of bed in the morning and was slightly breathless. Dr Obi visited in the early evening. She noted that David had been diagnosed with a viral illness and that although his vomiting had settled he still had a headache, his whole body ached, his cough was slightly worse and he felt breathless. Dr Obi measured his pulse, blood pressure and oxygen saturation. These were 70/min, 130/70 mmHg and 92% respectively. Dr Obi listened to his chest, which was normal. She explained that it was common to feel so achy with 'flu and that there was no evidence that he had a chest infection. Dr Obi explained that he would fight the infection himself and antibiotics would not be helpful.

David's condition deteriorated during the evening and his wife dialled 999 when he collapsed trying to get to the toilet. The ambulance arrived 10 minutes later but resuscitation was unsuccessful.

The cause of death at postmortem was bronchopneumonia.

It was alleged that Dr Jumali and Dr Obi failed to appreciate how unwell David was and that they failed to make an adequate assessment.

Do you think his claim will succeed?

 Expert comment

Death due to pneumonia in a patient aged 42 without pre-existing risk factors that compromise his/her immunity (such as HIV infection or cystic fibrosis) is very rare indeed.

A national confidential enquiry into community acquired pneumonia deaths in young adults in England and Wales found 27 deaths from community acquired pneumonia (CAP) in previously fit adults aged 15–44 in England and Wales in a one year period from September 1995. This is an incidence of 1.2 per million per year in this age group (Simpson *et al.*, 2000).

Two key questions in this case are whether it was possible to diagnose David's pneumonia and if the doctors who saw him recorded sufficient detail to demonstrate that they performed an adequate assessment.

It is well recognized that there are no symptoms or signs that 'rule in' the diagnosis of pneumonia (Metlay *et al.*, 1997). The diagnosis is often made on clinical grounds. However there is poor internal consistency between the auscultatory findings of different physicians and poor correlation between those findings and X-ray evidence of pneumonia (Wipf *et al.*, 1999).

The cardinal signs of pneumonia are (Metlay *et al.*, 1997; Hooker *et al.*, 1989):
- A temperature of over 37.8 °C
- A heart rate over 100 bpm
- A raised respiratory rate (tachypnoea)– normal rate at rest 16 to 25 breaths/minute.
- Crackles in the chest on auscultation.

Fever, raised respiratory rate and tachycardia are commonly present in acute bronchitis. Most studies

Avoiding Errors in General Practice, First Edition. Kevin Barraclough, Jenny du Toit, Jeremy Budd, Joseph E. Raine, Kate Williams and Jonathan Bonser.
© 2013 John Wiley & Sons, Ltd. Published 2013 by John Wiley & Sons, Ltd.

indicate that if the clinician makes a clinical diagnosis of pneumonia it is only confirmed on chest X-ray in 13% to 39% of cases (Metlay *et al.*, 1997).

Although it is well recognized that these clinical features may be absent in the elderly who have pneumonia (McFadden *et al.*, 1982), most practising clinicians would expect them to be present in a younger person with pneumonia. The updated British Thoracic Society guidelines in 2009 on Community Acquired Pneumonia (BTS, 2009) cites studies which suggest that the absence of abnormal vital signs and a clear chest on auscultation excludes the possibility of pneumonia to a high level of probability. This is an example of a 'SNOUT' (if a high Sensitivity clinical feature (the presence of abnormal vital signs or chest signs) is Negative it rules the diagnosis OUT). Therefore the common belief would be that, in the absence of fever, tachycardia and a raised respiratory rate, pneumonia can be effectively excluded as a possibility.

Pulse oximetry is being used more frequently in primary care. One study of 664 healthy volunteers and patients of mean age 50.6 years who had pulse oximetry and arterial blood gases measured for the purposes of the study found that the mean pulse oximetry measurement was 92.2% and the standard deviation was 6.4%. 29% of the study population had a pulse oximetry level below 90% (Lee *et al.*, 2000). The place of pulse oximetry in the assessment of CAP in primary care is not yet clear. The Primary Care Respiratory Society guidelines on the management of CAP in the community state that 'A low oxygen saturation of < 90%, especially in young patients without chronic lung disease, supports a decision to refer to hospital' (PCRS, 2010).

There is considerable pressure on general practitioners to avoid prescribing antibiotics in uncomplicated respiratory tract infections (Macfarlane *et al.*, 2001) (this is referred to as 'antibiotic stewardship' (Hooker, 1989)) but antibiotics are required treatment for CAP (BTS, 2001, 2009). However while other infections presenting as acute cough, such as acute bronchitis or rhinosinusitis, may respond to antibiotics, the only acute respiratory infection in which delayed treatment with antibiotics has been shown to increase the risk of death is pneumonia (Metlay & Fine, 2003).

Once the diagnosis of (probable) pneumonia is made in the community the general practitioner has to decide whether or not the patient requires admission to hospital. Most CAP is managed in the community and the condition does not usually require confirmation of the diagnosis with a chest X-ray (BTS, 2001, 2009). Most patients with pneumonia who are at low risk can be

treated with a broad spectrum antibiotic such as amoxicillin (BTS, 2001, 2009). Only patients who are at increased risk of death or serious complications require admission to hospital (BTS, 2001, 2009). CRB-65 'rule' (BTS, 2001, 2009) defines those at high risk:
- confusion
- raised respiratory rate ($\geq$ 30/min)
- low blood pressure (< 90/ $\leq$ 60)
- aged $\geq$ 65 years.

Neither Dr Jumali nor Dr Obi recorded a complete assessment of David. Even if Dr Jumali did ask about respiratory symptoms he has not documented the fact. Dr Obi recorded the fact that David's cough had worsened and that he was breathless. However she did not clarify the features of David's breathlessness nor record other symptoms such as chest pain, sputum or haemoptysis. The presence or absence of confusion is not recorded but it is likely that had this been present the doctors would have noted it. Nether general practitioner recorded David's respiratory rate. The oxygen saturation measured by Dr Obi was not low enough to alert her to the need to consider admitting David to hospital.

In her witness statement David's wife said that he was extremely unwell and very breathless.

If an adequate history and examination had been recorded and there were no fever, tachycardia, tachypnoea or chest signs then it would be possible to defend Dr Jumali and Dr Obi's actions. The outcome of cases often ends up being determined by whether the Court prefers the account of Claimant or the Defendant as to what features were present at what time. That is one reason why good quality notes are usually helpful to the general practitioner.

 Legal comment

Dr Jumali found none of the four cardinal signs of pneumonia. The potential weakness for his defence is that although he did examine the respiratory system, his notes do not mention the respiration rate. He will probably say that if the respiration rate had been high, he would have noticed and recorded it.

Dr Obi noted that David felt breathless, but again did not record the respiration rate. Nor does she record any temperature. She is likely to say the same. Both doctors are likely to say they found nothing to indicate catastrophic illness.

David's wife, on the other hand, says he was extremely unwell and very breathless. However, it is interesting to note that the Out of Hours service records her as saying at the time that he was 'slightly breathless'.

This is a case which the lawyers may well wish to defend at least at first. After all, the two doctors present similar accounts and the illness is extremely rare. A final decision on whether to defend or settle the case will probably be made after expert reports have been exchanged and after the experts have met to discuss the case.

As an accountant, David may well have been a high earner. The claim will be expensive, if it needs to be settled.

 Key learning points

Specific to the case
- Death due to pneumonia in a previously fit young adult is rare.
- When assessing a patient with symptoms suggestive of a chest infection it is essential to measure and record the temperature pulse and blood pressure.
- The place of pulse oximetry in the assessment of CAP still needs to be defined.

General points
- It is essential to record an assessment that allows the consultation to be reconstructed and provides the salient features on which management decisions should be based.

References

BTS (2001) Guidelines for the management of community acquired pneumonia in adults. *Thorax* **56**: 1iv–64

BTS (2009) Guidelines for the management of community acquired pneumonia in adults: 2009 update. *Thorax* **64**: 1–55.

Hooker E, O'Brien D, Danzi DF, Barefoot JAC, Brown JE (1989) Respiratory rates in emergency department patients. *Journal of Emergency Medicine* **7**: 129–32.

Lee WW, Mayberry K, Crapo R, Jensen RL (2000) The accuracy of pulse oximetry in the emergency department. *The American Journal of Emergency Medicine* **18**: 427–31.

Macfarlane J, Holmes W, Gard P, Macfarlane R, Rose D, Weston V *et al.* (2001) Prospective study of the incidence, aetiology and outcome of adult lower respiratory tract illness in the community. *Thorax* **56**: 109–14.

McFadden J, Price RC, Eastwood HD, Briggs RS (1982) Raised respiratory rate in elderly patients: a valuable physical sign. *BMJ* **284**: 626–7.

Metlay JP, Kapoor WN, Fine MJ (1997) Does this patient have community-acquired pneumonia? Diagnosing pneumonia by history and physical examination. *JAMA* **278**:1440–5.

Metlay JP, Fine MJ (2003) Testing strategies in the initial management of patients with community-acquired pneumonia. *Annals of Internal Medicine* **138**: 109–18.

PCRS (2010) Primary Care Respiratory Society UK – Opinion No. 33.

Simpson JCG, Macfarlane JT, Watson J, Woodhead MA (2000) A national confidential enquiry into community acquired pneumonia deaths in young adults in England and Wales. *Thorax* **55**: 1040–5.

Wipf JE, Lipsky BA, Hirschmann JV, Boyko EJ, *et al.* (1999) *Archives of Internal Medicine* **159**: 1082–7.

Case 26 Lost prescription: Benzodiazepine addiction

Samantha was 26. She arrived in reception at her GP surgery. She requested a prescription for diazepam tablets 5 mg, in a dose of two tablets three times a day, for a month. The same prescription had been issued 10 days earlier. The patient explained that she had just returned from a week's holiday in Ibiza and had unfortunately left her tablets behind in her hotel room.

Dr Balla, the GP registrar who was on duty that day used the patient's contact telephone number to speak to her. Samantha assured Dr Balla that her story was true and said she had previously had an epileptic fit when she had run out of tablets. Dr Balla issued the prescription.

A few days later Dr Balla was very upset to be contacted by the police. Samantha had been arrested for dealing in various drugs including diazepam. The police wanted to interview Dr Balla about the prescription. They said that under Section 29 of the Data Protection Act, she was entitled to release information without the parent's consent.

Careful examination of the prescribing records indicated Samantha had ordered and been prescribed 15 monthly increments of her prescription in the last year, and had also obtained an additional issue from the Out of Hours service a few months previously by stating that she had arrived too late at the GP surgery to collect her prescription.

What options were open to the GP?

Samantha was plausible and Dr Balla was deceived. She had also felt pressured by the story of an epileptic fit.

At the time the request was made, Dr Balla could have reviewed the previous ordering pattern and would have discovered the over-ordering. However, she was not responsible for the continuing prescription, or the lack of previous medication review, or lack of response to the Out of Hours incident.

Should she speak to the police?

 Expert comment

Benzodiazepine prescribing remains very common in general practice, despite the recommendation in the British National Formulary that all the drugs should only be given for short courses if being used to treat anxiety and insomnia. Over 12 million prescriptions for benzodiazepine are still dispensed annually in the UK.

Many benzodiazepines have a definite 'street value' and so diversion for criminal purposes is a significant risk.

Addiction and abuse of benzodiazepines also remains a significant problem and it remains one of the commonest causes of litigation against GPs, with patients alleging that they have suffered long term mental and physical health problems.

Warning signs include dose escalation; presenting too early for repeat prescriptions; abuse of other drugs; and stories of lost tablets, lost FP10s, and third parties stealing or throwing the tablets away.

Various strategies may be used. Diazepam can be prescribed using blue FP10 (instalment dispensing forms). Prescriptions may be issued weekly, with screen messages to prevent early ordering. Patients may be warned that stories of lost tablets will not be accepted.

 Legal comment

A doctor owes his patients a duty of confidentiality in law and in ethics. Breach of that duty is a serious matter, which can lead to sanctions by the GMC. However, the duty is not absolute. For example, statute requires that doctors notify certain authorities of known or suspected cases of certain communicable diseases. This is just one example of how the wider public interest in

Avoiding Errors in General Practice, First Edition. Kevin Barraclough, Jenny du Toit, Jeremy Budd, Joseph E. Raine, Kate Williams and Jonathan Bonser.
© 2013 John Wiley & Sons, Ltd. Published 2013 by John Wiley & Sons, Ltd.

disclosure can outweigh the advantages of maintaining confidentiality.

The GMC puts the principle like this:

> Personal information may therefore be disclosed in the public interest without the patient's consent, and in exceptional cases where patients have withheld consent, if the benefits to an individual or to society of the disclosure outweigh both the public and the patient's interest in keeping the information confidential.

Dr Balla needs to have this principle in mind when considering the police's request for information about Samantha's prescription. They have quoted the Data Protection Act to her in support of their request. But this Act is only concerned with whether or not data is processed fairly. It does not cover her legal and professional duties of confidentiality.

So Dr Balla has to do a balancing exercise between the interests of her patient and the public interest in the prevention and detection of crime. This is how the GMC puts it:

> You must weigh the harms that are likely to arise from non-disclosure of information against the possible harm both to the patient and to the overall trust between doctors and patients arising from the release of that information.

The first step for Dr Balla to take is to ask for Samantha's permission to disclose the records. If she says no, then the balancing exercise has to be done. In this case, Dr Balla may feel some embarrassment about having issued the prescriptions. That might affect her judgement. These balancing exercises are difficult enough in the best of circumstances. So she should definitely take advantage of the expertise available through her MDO. A medico-legal adviser will talk through the case and help Dr Balla reach an objective and considered decision.

She may conclude that she cannot see clearly enough who might be harmed if the information is not disclosed. If she declines to share the information with the police, then they will have the option of seeking a court order requiring the disclosure. At that point, Dr Balla will have no choice but to comply unless she has some grave concern about the consequences for her patient. In that case, she needs to get back in touch with her MDO.

If she decides the balance is in favour of making the disclosure to the police, then she needs to carefully record how she came to that decision. In principle, Samantha could either sue Dr Balla for breaching her confidence or report her to the GMC. But if Dr Balla can show that she took care to make a balanced judgement, then she will be able to defend herself successfully.

 Key learning points

Specific to the case
- The request for an unscheduled benzodiazepine prescription should be considered carefully in the light of the prescribing history.

General points
- It is wise to seek advice from your defence organization before divulging any confidential information to the police.

Further reading

Ashton H (2005) The diagnosis and management of benzodiazepine dependence. *Current Opinion in Psychiatry* **18**: 249–55.

British National Formulary – sections on anxiolytics and hypnotics

General Medical Council (2009) Guidance on 'Confidentiality'. GMC.

Case 27 A febrile baby

Emma had an uneventful birth. At the age of six months she was taken to the doctor by her mother, Susan. Susan was worried because Emma was 'burning up' and snuffly. She said that Emma was not feeding well, was making funny noises when she breathed and had a rash.

Dr Moore saw Emma. His clinical note detailed that the baby was unwell and had been tachypnoeic that day. He noted that Emma was drinking but not taking solids.

What features would you have specifically noted?

On examination he recorded that Emma felt hot but was alert. He made a tick after fontanelle, throat, ears, chest and abdomen and indicated that there was no photophobia or neck stiffness. He diagnosed a viral illness, advised calpol and fluids and that Emma should be seen again if she got worse.

Would you have done anything differently?

Early the next morning Susan contacted the Out of Hours (OOH) service because Emma has been irritable during the night. Susan had gone to check on Emma and found that she was drowsy and had a purple rash. The OOH Service advised Susan to call an ambulance. A visiting doctor also went but by the time they arrived Emma had already been taken to hospital. On admission a diagnosis of meningococcal septicaemia was made. Unfortunately Emma suffered brain damage and was severely handicapped as a result of her illness.

Susan felt that Dr Moore should have referred Emma to hospital as an emergency. Dr Moore was sued for alleged negligence.

Do you think his claim will succeed?

 ## Expert comment

The suspicion of meningococcal meningitis or septicaemia is a challenge for general practitioners for several reasons:

- The condition is rare. A full time general practitioner is only likely to see one or two cases in their career. The diagnosis is suspected from text book descriptions and the recognition that the patient is generally unwell.
- The early features are the same as those of minor viral illness. A 2006 paper in *The Lancet* showed that by 20–22 hours after the onset of the illness only 50% of children under the age of one had developed features of septicaemia, only 30% had a haemorrhagic rash and only 20% had impaired consciousness (Thompson *et al.*, 2006).
- The condition may get rapidly worse. It is not uncommon for a doctor to have seen a patient a few hours before and not realized the severity of the illness. In one study the researchers examined 177 cases of meningococcal disease retrospectively (Toft Sorenson *et al.*, 1992). Of these 92 (52%) had seen a doctor who had not recognized the likelihood of serious disease in the period immediately prior to admission.

The Meningitis Trust was established in 1986 following a prolonged outbreak of meningococcal disease in Stroud and Stonehouse, Gloucestershire. This helped to improve both public and medical awareness of the disease. Information leaflets were distributed throughout the county highlighting features of the condition: a distinctive haemorrhagic rash (which could be recognized as nonblanching by the 'tumbler test'), impaired consciousness, a stiff neck and, in infants, a bulging fontanelle and a high-pitched scream. Thompson *et al.* (2006) highlighted the fact that the 'classical' features

Avoiding Errors in General Practice, First Edition. Kevin Barraclough, Jenny du Toit, Jeremy Budd, Joseph E. Raine, Kate Williams and Jonathan Bonser.
© 2013 John Wiley & Sons, Ltd. Published 2013 by John Wiley & Sons, Ltd.

of the disease occur very late. They advocated looking for certain earlier features of the disease (such as cold peripheries, a mottled discolouration of the skin and limb pains).

In the past many general practitioners would have made an assessment like that made by Dr Williams. This gave a general impression of the clinical condition of a child. However he has omitted some details that would have given a clearer picture not only at the time but subsequently when the case was being scrutinized.

NICE (2007) published guidance on the assessment and initial management of feverish illness in children under 5 years. This gives a traffic light system for assessing the severity of illness. Children with 'Red' features should be admitted urgently, children with 'amber' features can either be managed at home with suitable 'safety netting' or admitted to hospital. These features provide a minimum data set that it would be helpful to record.

1. General comments re colour, level consciousness, feeding and urine output.
2. Temperature. In the era of mercury thermometers general practitioners often did not record a temperature. There is reasonable evidence that assessment of the presence of fever by touch (fever defined as a temperature over 37.8 °C or 38 °C) is sensitive (it detects most children with fever) but poorly specific (it incorrectly identifies afebrile children as febrile) (Buckley & Conine, 1996; Hung *et al.*, 2000; Whybrew *et al.*, 1998). Nowadays an aural thermometer should always be used to record the temperature of a child.
3. Heart rate. Although it is advisable to measure heart rate, NICE (2007) found a lack of evidence that heart rate was a marker of serious disease. One difficulty is that the 'normal range' of heart rate changes significantly in the first year of life. A second difficulty is that the 'normal range', particularly with fever, is not well defined.
4. Respiratory rate. Nasal flaring, grunting and intercostal and subcostal recession are markers of respiratory distress. Margolis & Gadornski (1998) concluded that 'The best individual finding for ruling out pneumonia is the absence of tachypnoea.' However it can be difficult to measure the respiratory rate in a febrile infant. The average respiratory rate of a one-week-old child is 50/min (per minute) and it falls to 40/min at 6 months. Fever elevates the respiratory rate by about 10/min per degree centigrade elevation in children without pneumonia (Margolis & Garornski, 1998). Furthermore, a young infant's respiratory rate is often very irregular when the child

is awake and being examined. It is best to measure the rate for 1 minute or two separate 30 second periods.

5. An assessment of hydration to include CRT and tissue turgor.
6. General features, in particular if there is bulging of the anterior fontanelle, rash or evidence of meningism.

Emma had one NICE amber feature, feeding poorly. She felt hot so probably had a raised temperature. If her fever had been <39 °C Dr William's action fell within the normal range. He did not feel that Emma's condition merited admission but provided safety netting.

His record of the safety netting was brief 'see if gets worse'. His advice to Susan needed to have detailed precisely what to look for, what to do if these things occurred, who to contact out of hours and follow up arrangements. It does appear that he did this because Susan contacted the Out of Hours service when Emma was drowsy and had a purple rash.

Dr Williams had written 'tachypnoeic that day' but he had also written 'chest √'. Dr Williams maintained that Emma had been breathing normally when he saw her. Susan disputed this and said that Emma had been breathing quickly, was snuffly and made funny noises when she breathed. Susan felt that because of her breathing difficulties Dr Williams should have admitted Emma to hospital. Although Dr Williams notes indicate that he did not feel Emma had respiratory distress, it would have been helpful if he had recorded the respiratory rate.

 Legal comment

According to Dr Williams's evidence, it appears that his care of Emma was reasonable. Based on his version of events, the case should be defensible. However, there are two potential areas of weakness and dispute: Emma's respiratory rate and the standard of safety netting. The lawyers will pick over Dr Williams's notes. In particular, they will home in on 'chest √' and 'see if get worse'. What *were* his findings? What *was* his advice? Based on Susan's evidence, her GP expert may conclude that Dr Williams should have admitted Emma.

In terms of causation, a paediatrician will have to comment on what would have happened at hospital. However, it is likely that the illness would have been diagnosed and treated in time. The causation experts may well, therefore, conclude that if Dr Williams had admitted Emma, she would not now be severely handicapped.

This case will be worth several million pounds in damages. How it is resolved will largely depend on the relative strengths of Dr Williams's and Susan's evidence.

Key learning points

Specific to the case
- Menigococcal disease is rare.
- Early signs of meningococcal infection are similar to those of minor self-limiting illness and it is often not possible to suspect the condition if the infant/child is seen close to the onset of the condition. It is therefore essential to provide detailed safety netting in any consultation with a febrile infant or child.

General point
- It is not uncommon for there to be a dispute about facts. A good clinical record is invaluable in these circumstances.

Further reading and references

Buckley R, Conine M (1996) Reliability of subjective fever in the triage of adult patients. *Annals of Emergency Medicine* **27**: 693–7.

Flemming S, Thompson M, *et al.* (2011) Normal ranges of heart rate and respiratory rate in children from birth to 18 years of age: a systematic review of observational studies. *Lancet* **377**: 1011–18.

Hung OL, Kwon NS, Cole AE, Dacpano GR, Wu T, Chiang WK *et al.* (2000) Evaluation of the physician's ability to recognize the presence or absence of anemia, fever, and jaundice. *Acad Emerg Med* **7**: 146–56.

Margolis P, Gadornski A (1998) Does this infant have pneumonia? *JAMA* **279**: 308–13.

NICE (2007) Feverish illness in children: Assessment and initial management in children younger than 5 years. NICE CG 47.

Thompson MJ, Ninis N, Perera R, Mayon-White R, Phillips C, Bailey L, *et al.* (2006) Clinical recognition of meningococcal disease in children and adolescents. *The Lancet* **367**: 397–403.

Toft Sorensen H, Moller-Petersen J, Bygum Krarup H, Pedersen H, Hansen H, Hamburger H (1992) Diagnostic problems with meningococcal disease in general practice. *Journal of Clinical Epidemiology* **45**: 1289–93.

Whybrew K, Murray M, Morley C (1998) Diagnosing fever by touch: observational study. *BMJ* **317**: 321–30.

Case 28 A limping elderly woman after a fall

May was a 79-year-old clerk. Three years previously she had had a right total hip replacement for osteoarthritis. Whilst visiting her daughter in France she had tripped in the garden and landed awkwardly on her left hip. Following the fall she was able to walk, although her left hip was rather painful. May found the journey home rather difficult and on her return requested a home visit because of the pain and bruising of her hip.

Dr Ali called later that day. Dr Ali noted that on examination there was bruising over the left buttock and that the left hip was tender. May was able to walk using a stick. The range of movement of the left hip was normal and there was no shortening or external rotation of the left leg. Dr Ali did not think that May had done any serious damage to herself but that the fall might have caused a flare of osteoarthritis.

May was still in a lot of pain a week later. She contacted the surgery and spoke to Dr Ali who prescribed some co-dydramol because the paracetamol and ibuprofen May had tried was not providing any relief.

Ten days later another home visit was requested. May did not feel well and had taken to her bed. Dr Grant elicited a history suggestive of a UTI. May did not look unwell and had a normal temperature, pulse and blood pressure. Dr Grant prescribed trimethoprim and asked May to contact the surgery if her symptoms did not settle over the next week. May also asked Dr Grant about her hip. It was still painful and she still had to use a stick. On examination the hip was 'normal'. Dr Grant thought that May had lost confidence and suggested referring May to physiotherapy.

Would you have done anything differently?

May was seen by the physiotherapist two weeks later. Initially her hip pain and walking seemed to improve. However on her third visit to the physiotherapist she stumbled as she left the department. The pain in her hip was much worse that night and she contacted the

surgery. Dr Ali visited May again. He noted that she was still getting pain weight bearing and that the pain was worse after stumbling the previous day. Dr Ali referred May for an X-ray that was done two days later. This showed an impacted sub-capital fracture of the left femur. May was admitted from X-ray and had a left total hip replacement.

It was alleged that the actions of the general practitioners were negligent in that they should have referred May for an X-ray earlier.

Do you think her claim will succeed?

 Expert comment

In retrospect May fractured her left neck of femur when she fell in France. It is also clear that when she was assessed by Dr Ali she was able to walk, weight bear and had a full range of hip movement.

Fractures of the femur are common in the elderly, particularly in women because of their low peak bone mass and accelerated bone loss for four to five years after menopause. There are 70 000–75 000 hip fractures annually in the UK and this is the commonest reason for admission to an orthopaedic ward (NICE, 2011). The average age of sustaining a fracture is 77 (NICE, 2011). Delay in surgical treatment has been shown to adversely affect rehabilitation (Villar *et al.*, 1986).

Usually a patient is unable to weight bear following a hip fracture. On examination the affected leg is shortened and externally rotated. Active and passive movements of the hip are extremely painful and limited. However, occasionally an elderly patient sustains an impacted, undisplaced fracture. In these circumstances the diagnosis is often delayed because there are no clinical signs (Williams *et al.*, 1984; McRae, 1981; Aston & Hughes, 1983).

One study of 1108 consecutive patients at Peterborough General Hospital with fractured neck of femur

Avoiding Errors in General Practice, First Edition. Kevin Barraclough, Jenny du Toit, Jeremy Budd, Joseph E. Raine, Kate Williams and Jonathan Bonser.
© 2013 John Wiley & Sons, Ltd. Published 2013 by John Wiley & Sons, Ltd.

found that the diagnosis was delayed for more than 24 hours in 154 patients (14%) (Pathak *et al.*, 1997). In 91 of the cases of delay the patient had been seen by a doctor (either in A&E or their general practitioner) and the fracture was not suspected. In another study the diagnosis of a hip fracture was delayed in 10% of cases (Eastwood, 1987). In this study elderly care physicians and general practitioners had often made an alternative diagnosis such as a flare of osteoarthritis and had not X-rayed the patient.

These and other studies indicate that delayed diagnosis of clinically 'occult' hip fractures in the elderly is not uncommon.

Current data suggests that significant falls occur annually in 35% of those aged 75 or over (Tinetti *et al.*, 1988). Of these 6% have fractures. A study in Newcastle found that, in one year, 4% of patients aged over 65 requested an ambulance because of falls (Newton *et al.*, 2006).

To avoid the delay in diagnosis it would be necessary to carry out X-rays in all elderly patients who have a history of fall whether or not they have clinical signs of a fracture. If such a recommendation were followed it would result in huge numbers of X-rays because falls are very common indeed in the elderly.

This raises a number of issues:

- There are often significant logistical difficulties of requesting X-rays in these circumstances. It is often necessary to request an ambulance because the elderly often do not have means of transport even if they are mobile.
- Hip and pelvic X-rays do carry a significant radiation dose with them (approximately equivalent to between 15 and 35 chest X-rays).
- It would also impose an enormous load on secondary care services.

The guidance document: *Making the Best Use of a Department of Clinical Radiology* was produced by the Royal College of Radiologists. This document recommends (4th Edition, 1998, recommendation D18, p. 43) that X-rays for hip pain when there is a full range of movement are not routinely indicated. (It is not clear whether a history of fall is considered to be significant with this recommendation.)

To assess whether a practice of X-raying all elderly patients with significant falls would be reasonable, it would be necessary to consider how many X-rays would need to be carried out to detect one clinically occult fracture in these circumstances (a sort of 'NNT').

In this case although May had had a fall she was able to walk and had managed the journey home. Dr

Ali made and recorded a full history and examination. May had no features to suggest a fractured neck of femur.

Given his findings the previous week it was entirely reasonable for Dr Ali to provide a prescription over the telephone a week later.

When Dr Grant visited May had features consistent of a UTI that were appropriately assessed and treated. He also examined the hip which was 'normal' although it would have been helpful for his defence if more details of the examination had been recorded. Many general practitioners would have organized physiotherapy as Dr Grant did. Some general practitioners may have organized an X-ray at this stage.

When Dr Ali visited May after she stumbled in the physiotherapy department he did not document an examination of the hip. Given the history of worse pain following a stumble having had a previous fall Dr Ali should have referred May for an X-ray that day if examination of the hip was not normal. He referred her for an X-ray which was performed two days later. The fracture was impacted and a two-day delay, if such it was, would not have had any consequences.

 Legal comment

Based on the expert opinion above, the case seems defensible. Dr Ali's and Dr Grant's treatment of May was appropriate up until Dr Ali's final visit, when he perhaps should have arranged an X-ray that day. However, even if his treatment was substandard in this regard, the delay of two days would have made no difference: May would still have required the hip replacement.

However, the lawyers representing May will undoubtedly question the telephone call, when May reported that ibuprofen and paracetamol were not relieving her pain. They will ask their GP expert whether Dr Ali should have visited May. Even if they conclude that he should have done, Dr Ali can defend himself by pointing to Dr Grant's later examination. But there are question marks over Dr Grant's home visit. We do not know how carefully he examined May's hip. May was in bed with what appeared to be a UTI. Did Dr Grant ask her to get out of bed and weight-bear?

If May's GP expert criticizes these earlier consultations, then orthopaedic experts will need to comment on what difference intervention would have made at those times: would May have been spared her left total hip replacement? If she would have needed the hip replacement anyway, then damages will be limited to a small figure representing pain and suffering during the period when the condition went undiagnosed: at most a little over a thousand pounds.

The lawyers for May will also wish to investigate the liability of the physiotherapist. Perhaps she should have recognized a problem earlier?

 Key learning points

Specific to the case
- If hip pain persists following a fall in an elderly person always consider the possibility of an impacted fracture of the neck of femur even if the hip appears to be 'normal'.

General points
- It is always necessary to make and record a further full assessment of a condition if symptoms persist beyond the duration to be expected.

References and further reading

Aston JN, Hughes S (1983) *Aston's Short Textbook of Orthopaedics and Tramatology*, 3rd Edition. Hodder &Stoughton, p. 106.

Brunner LC, Eshilian-Oates L, Kuo TY (2003) Hip fractures in adults. *American Family Physician* **67**(3): 537–42. Available at www.aafp.org/afp

Eastwood HDH (1987) Delayed diagnosis of femoral-neck fractures in the elderly. *Age and Ageing* **16**(16): 378–82.

McRae R (1981) *Practical Fracture Treatment*. Churchill Livingstone, p. 217.

Newton JL, Kyle P, Liversidge P, Robinson G, Wilton K, Reeve P (2006) The costs of falls in the community to the North East Ambulance Service. *Emerg Med J* 2006;**23**:479-81.

NICE (2011) The management of hip fracture in adults. CG 124.

Pathak G, Parker MJ, Pryor GA (1997). Delayed diagnosis of femoral neck fractures. *Injury* **28**: 299–301.

Tinetti ME, Speechley M, Ginter SF (1988) Risk factors for falls among elderly persons living in the community. *N Engl J Med* **319**: 1701–7.

Villar RN, Allen SM, Barnes SJ (1986) Hip fractures in healthy patients: operative delay versus prognosis. *BMJ* **293**: 1203.

Williams NS, Bulstrode CJK, O'Connell PR (1984) *Bailey and Love's Short Practice of Surgery*, 19th Edition. H.K. Lewis & Co., p. 283.

Case 29 Indigestion in a stressed executive

Malcolm was a 46-year-old senior banking executive in the City who had a BMI of 37 and smoked. When he consulted Dr Mathers it was usually in order to request a private referral to a named specialist whom a colleague or friend had recommended. He always appeared rushed and tended to dominate consultations. On this occasion he saw Dr Mathers and asked for a referral to a back specialist whose details he supplied. Dr Mathers noticed that the last recorded blood pressure was 5 years earlier and a letter from an occupational health assessment had noted a blood pressure of 190/110 mmHg 2 years earlier. Dr Mathers checked his blood pressure and noted it was 170/104 mmHg. He asked Malcolm to have his blood pressure checked twice further by the nurse and have blood tests and an ECG. However, Malcolm did not attend for another 7 months.

On the next occasion Malcolm consulted Dr Mathers he was not sleeping, sweating a lot and had been getting burning retrosternal chest discomfort at night. He sometimes felt breathless. Malcolm was extremely stressed because his department had lost a great deal of money and he was being held responsible. Dr Mathers noted that he had consulted the Out of Hours service two weeks earlier with dysuria, was noted to have microscopic haematuria and had been treated with an antibiotic. Dr Mathers noted that chest examination was normal but his blood pressure was 184/112 mmHg.

What would you do now?

Dr Mathers arranged for Malcolm to have an ECG with the nurse. This was normal. He prescribed amlodipine 5 mg daily and omeprazole 20 mg daily, arranged for Malcolm to have some routine blood tests and referred him for a private cardiology opinion.

What would be your differential diagnosis have been and how would you discriminate between them?

Unfortunately, 4 days later Malcolm was found dead in bed by his wife. His wife said that he had been complaining of chest pains and breathlessness for several days. At post mortem he had widespread coronary atheroma, no myocardial infarction but a grossly hypertrophied and dilated heart with extensive myocardial fibrosis. There was also pulmonary oedema and congestion.

His wife brought an action against Dr Mathers and the practice for failing to adequately monitor or treat Malcolm's blood pressure and for failing to recognize symptoms of myocardial ischaemia.

Do you think his claim will succeed?

 Expert comment

The assessment of chest pain continues to cause problems for general practitioners and cases of sudden cardiac death, missed heart failure and myocardial infarction continue to be common causes of litigation. One difficulty is that chest pain is very common. A fulltime general practitioner can expect to see a new case every one to two weeks. Musculoskeletal chest pain and gastro oesophageal reflux (GORD) are very common causes – but stable angina, unstable angina and myocardial infarction are also not rare. A particular diagnostic problem is when there is a history of chest pain but the patient has not got chest pain at the time of the assessment.

In this case, as is often the case, there was a problem for Dr Mathers' defence because the characteristics of

Avoiding Errors in General Practice, First Edition. Kevin Barraclough, Jenny du Toit, Jeremy Budd, Joseph E. Raine, Kate Williams and Jonathan Bonser.
© 2013 John Wiley & Sons, Ltd. Published 2013 by John Wiley & Sons, Ltd.

the chest pain were not well documented. In particular, there were no details about how long the chest pains had been occurring, how frequently they occurred, how long the episodes lasted and whether they were related to exertion or not. It was also not clear if the episodes of breathlessness were associated in time with the chest pains or not.

An additional problem was that the purpose of the ECG was not clear from Dr Mather's clinical note. If it was to exclude angina or an acute coronary syndrome then it was clearly unsafe.

In March 2010 the UK's National Institute of Clinical Excellence (NICE) produced guidance on the Assessment of Chest Pain of Recent Onset (CG 95).

The guidance points out that it is generally safe and reasonable to exclude a diagnosis of stable angina if the characteristics of the pain are non-anginal. Typical anginal pain has three characteristics. It is:

1. retrosternal,
2. brought on by exertion, and
3. relieved by rest.

'Atypical angina' is chest pain with two of these three characteristics. Non-anginal chest pain has one or none of these features.

However, most of the diagnostic difficulties that result in medico-legal cases occur in cases of 'acute coronary syndrome' (ACS). This group comprises what used to be called myocardial infarction and unstable angina. It seems to be the latter group – unstable angina – that causes the diagnostic problems. The patient with chest pain at the time of assessment appears to be assessed quite well and patients are usually sent urgently for full assessment to A&E. In medico-legal cases it seems to be unstable angina that is relatively poorly recognized.

The NICE guidance is helpful up to a point. If 'ACS suspected' and the last pain was within 12 hours, do an ECG and if abnormal in any way (including nonspecific findings such as abnormal T wave inversion) then treat as ACS (aspirin, oxygen stats etc.) and admit urgently to hospital via '999' ambulance. If the ECG is completely normal, or the last chest pain was more than 12 hours earlier then refer for same day hospital assessment. If the last chest pain was more than 72 hours ago then assess whether referral is necessary or needs to be urgent.

Of course the decision tree hangs on whether ACS is 'suspected'. In this case Malcolm, even on the basis of Dr Mathers' slightly scant recorded history, had recurrent retrosternal burning chest pain occurring at rest or at night. General practitioners often consider burning retrosternal pain to be likely to be due to GORD. However, in a UK study of 972 patients, average age 50, presenting to A&E with acute undifferentiated chest pain (a normal ECG and not obviously ACS for some other reason), 8% turned out to have ACS.

The independent predictors of ACS included burning pain (odds ratio 3), pain radiating into the arms, vomiting and smoking status (Goodacre *et al.*, 2003). A meta-analysis in the excellent Rational Clinical Examination series in *JAMA* noted that pain radiating into both arms was a strong predictor (Likelihood Ratio of 6) as was sweating (Panju *et al.*, 1998). Chest pain that was sharp (well localized in position and time), stabbing, positional or reproduced by palpation all markedly reduced the likelihood of a cardiac cause (likelihood ratios of around 0.2).

Allegations of failure to assess and treat hypertension adequately are also relatively common, particularly in the context of a younger patient who may have had a stroke. In this case, Malcolm was a rather dominating patient who tended to dictate the terms of his own care. This is not a mitigating factor. A general practitioner should insist on taking a full history. If the patient refuses to cooperate, then this should be noted. However, to say that Malcolm was overbearing is no defence.

The finding of microscopic haematuria in a male should have been followed up by the practice and repeated and investigated if persistent (Kelly *et al.*, 2009).

Overall, the claim is likely to succeed because Malcolm was a high risk individual for ACS (hypertensive, obese, smoker, male, 46) and had recurrent, unexplained and poorly documented retrosternal burning chest pains. Depending on whether the last episode of chest pain was more or less than 12 hours earlier he needed urgent admission or same day assessment for ACS.

 Legal comment

It will prove difficult to defend this case, if only because of the lack of detail in the medical records. A cardiologist will have to report on causation, but it is likely that earlier intervention would have saved Malcolm's life.

The claim will be expensive. The valuation will depend on what Malcolm's life expectancy would have been, if he had received timely treatment. The largest component of the damages will be based on Malcolm's earnings and banker's salaries and bonuses are notoriously high. If we assume that he would have lived until a retiring age of 65 and that he had an annual post tax pay of £200 000, then at full value, the case would be worth in excess of £2 000 000.

Key learning points

Specific to the case
- Stable angina can usually be identified or discarded as a possibility by three questions. Is the pain:
1. retrosternal,
2. brought on by exertion, and
3. relieved by rest.
- However, most medico-legal difficulties occur with the assessment of 'atypical angina' type pains (2 of the 3 factors above), or non-anginal pain (1 or none) occurring within the context of unstable angina. Typically the patient has no chest pain at the time of assessment and the 12 lead ECG is normal. The risk that the chest pain is cardiac in origin is probably of the order of 5% to 10% (in a UK A&E population) (Goodacre et al., 2003).
- Features that increase the likelihood that non-anginal chest pain may be cardiac (and therefore ACS) are as follows:
  ○ higher risk patient (age, male, risk factors such as smoking, hypertension, diabetes, hypercholesterolaemia);
  ○ retrosternal burning chest pain lasting more than 15 minutes;
  ○ chest pain radiating into one or both arms, or the neck;
  ○ nausea, vomiting or sweating.

- Factors that reduce the risk of ACS are chest pain that is (LR around 0.2):
  ○ sharp (well localized in position and time);
  ○ stabbing;
  ○ positional; or
  ○ reproduced by palpation.

General points
- It is important to stay up to date with key parts of clinical guidance that effect primary care such as the NICE guidance on the Assessment of Chest Pain of Recent Onset (CG 95).
- Microscopic haematuria in a male always requires follow up.

References and further reading

Goodacre SW, Angelini K, Arnold J, Revill S, Morris F (2003) Clinical predictors of acute coronary syndromes in patients with undifferentiated chest pain. *Quarterly Journal of Medicine* **96**: 893–8.

Kelly KD, Fawcett DP, Goldberg LC (200) Assessment and management of non-visible haematuria in primary care. *BMJ* **388**:bmj.a3021.

NICE (2010) NICE guidance on the Assessment of Chest Pain of Recent Onset. CG95.

Panju AA, Hemmelgarn BR, Guyatt GH, Simel DL (1998) Is this patient having a myocardial infarction? *JAMA* **280**: 1256–63.

Case 30 A hoped-for pregnancy

Celia was a 38-year-old woman who had had tubal surgery at the age of 33 after some years of subfertility. Unfortunately, despite the surgery she failed to conceive for many years. She was therefore delighted when she consulted Dr Anton with two sequential positive pregnancy tests and her LMP 6 weeks earlier.

What would you do now?

Dr Anton congratulated Celia, sent a urine sample for a hospital pregnancy test, referred Celia to the midwife and arranged to see her again in four weeks.

Three days later Dr Anton's colleague Dr Boulton received and reviewed the results of the pregnancy test (Dr Anton was on holiday). The hospital test was negative ('< 25 IU HCG/L'). Dr Boulton recorded that the urine sample had probably not been the first of the day. The following day Celia rang another GP at the surgery Dr Clarke and advised that she had had a little lower abdominal cramp but no vaginal bleeding. Dr Clarke advised her of the result of the test but suggested a repeat early morning urine sample to test and to see the midwife as planned but to report any further pain.

What would be your differential diagnosis and what would you do?

One week later Celia was admitted as an emergency via A&E in a collapsed state with an ectopic pregnancy. After an emergency laparotomy, salpingectomy and a transfusion of 6 units of blood Celia was discharged three weeks later.

Celia made a complaint to the practice that she had been told in the hospital that she should have been referred urgently for an ultrasound scan when she was pregnant because she was at such high risk of ectopic pregnancy. Dr Anton explained that there was nothing in the correspondence from the fertility clinic that had advised this course of action. Later Celia brought an action against Dr Anton and her colleagues for failure to refer her urgently for an ultrasound once it was realized she was pregnant.

Do you think her claim will succeed?

 ## Expert comment

Claims against general practitioners for alleged failures to diagnose or suspect ectopic pregnancies remain common. This is unsurprising since approximately 1 in 100 pregnancies are ectopic (1% risk).

A review article in *The Lancet* in 1998 gave risk factors for ectopic pregnancy (Pisarska *et al.*, 1998). The odds ratio (essentially equivalent to a likelihood ratio) was 21 with a past history of tubal surgery. This corresponds to an absolute risk of ectopic pregnancy of about 17.5% (21/120). NICE (2004) gave guidance on fertility assessment and treatment quotes research evidence for an ectopic rate of 23% per pregnancy in patients who underwent surgery for distal tubal occlusions and 8% who underwent surgery for proximal tubal occlusion. The odds ratio associated with past pelvic inflammatory disease is about 4.

This very high risk of ectopic pregnancy after tubal surgery does not appear to be widely publicized and there is no general guidance that advises urgent referral for an ultrasound to confirm that the pregnancy is intra uterine. Yet the very high risk of ectopic pregnancy in this situation would seem to indicate that urgent referral for an ultrasound when the woman is found to be pregnant is absolutely necessary.

There is no guidance that indicates that referral for ultrasound is uniform practice and many general practitioners may be unaware of the very high risk of ectopic pregnancy in cases such as Celia. At first impression, this would appear to offer Dr Anton a *Bolam* defence. Many competent general practitioners would be unaware of quite how high the risk of ectopic pregnancy is after tubal surgery. However, given the clear published

Avoiding Errors in General Practice, First Edition. Kevin Barraclough, Jenny du Toit, Jeremy Budd, Joseph E. Raine, Kate Williams and Jonathan Bonser.
© 2013 John Wiley & Sons, Ltd. Published 2013 by John Wiley & Sons, Ltd.

figures, a failure to refer appears unlikely to stand up to the logical scrutiny of the Court. Thus Dr Anton's treatment of Celia is likely to fail on the *Bolitho* test.

The specialist fertility clinic was also arguably at fault for failing to warn the general practitioners or Celia that an urgent ultrasound would be required if she became pregnant.

Dr Boulton appeared to be unaware that modern monoclonal antibody based urine tests (ELISA tests) brought in the late 1980s were far more sensitive and will detect βhCG at levels as low as 25 mIU/ml. This means pregnancy can be detected by two weeks after ovulation or four weeks after the last period (virtually by the time the next period would be due if the woman was not pregnant). It has not been necessary to have a concentrated early morning urine sample for many years. It is important that general practitioners keep up to date with the performance characteristics of tests they regularly use.

A urinary pregnancy test that reverts from being positive to being negative at six weeks is highly suggestive of a failed pregnancy. This could be due to an intra-uterine blighted ovum or it could be due to the implanted ovum failing because it is in an ectopic site. The negative pregnancy test was another indication that an urgent ultrasound was required to see if Celia had an intra-uterine pregnancy, or an ectopic one.

The last problem was that Dr Clarke appears not to have acted when notified about the presence of lower abdominal pain. Tay *et al.* (2000) put it succinctly:

Any sexually active woman presenting with abdominal pain and vaginal bleeding after a period of amenorrhea has an ectopic pregnancy until proved otherwise. Women who present in a collapsed state usually have had prodromal symptoms that have been overlooked. Tubal rupture is rarely sudden since it is due to invasion of the trophoblast. Therefore if there is any suspicion hospital referral for investigation is mandatory.

Once Celia had significant lower abdominal pain plus a positive pregnancy test (particularly as it had turned from positive to negative) it was essential that she was referred urgently into hospital.

It is often the case, as in this example, that the harm occurs because of a concatenation of errors by different individuals. Experts are often asked to advise on 'apportionment' in such cases – how much should each defendant (or, more usually, their MDO) pay.

If all three general practitioners are found to be in breach of duty (which would be likely in this case) their degree of liability (the fraction of the whole damages that their MDO has to pay) will be determined by relative degree of the Claimant's loss consequent upon each breach of duty. 'But for' each act Celia's loss (the collapse and need for urgent surgery) would have been avoided. If the case came to Court (which would be unlikely – see the legal comment) the damages would be split equally between the three general practitioners. It is the consequences of the individual breaches of duty that determines the apportionment of damages, rather than whether each action was a slip or a more serious error.

Legal comment

As mentioned above, it will prove difficult to defend Dr Anton's standard of care. Even if he can be defended in terms of the *Bolam* test, he will probably fail on the logical analysis demanded by the *Bolitho* test. The other defendant's would be equally liable.

But the value of the case will not be high. A gynaecological expert will conclude that Celia would have had to undergo the salpingectomy (or would have lost the use of the affected fallopian tube) in any event. She may have been saved the laparotomy; that is to say, the surgery perhaps could have been performed laparoscopically or medically. With earlier intervention, the surgery would have been earlier and she would have been saved several days pain. She would also probably have been discharged earlier. The damages will be limited to a few thousand pounds.

Key learning points

Specific to the case
- Ectopic pregnancy has to be considered as one of the 'must not miss' diagnoses in any woman of child-bearing age with abdominal pain or abnormal vaginal bleeding.
- In December 2001 The Chief Medical Officer pointed out that:

All clinicians, particular those working in primary care and Accident and Emergency Departments need to be aware of atypical clinical presentations of ectopic pregnancy...

Urinary dipstick testing for βhCG should be performed in any woman of reproductive age with unexplained abdominal pain. The test is now rapid, easy and sensitive...'

- An unexplained finding, such as a pregnancy test going from positive to negative, needs to be explained. In this case it was clear evidence that the ovum had failed, whether in an ectopic site or in utero.

General points

• It is important that general practitioners stay up to date with the performance characteristics of new tests that they frequently use.

• Even if a practice is widespread among general practitioners it may not be defensible in court if the practice does not stand up to logical scrutiny.

References and further reading

Jukovic D, Wilkinson H (2011) Diagnosis and management of ectopic pregnancy. *BMJ* **342**: d3397.

NICE (2004) *Fertility: Assessment and Treatment for People with Fertility Problems*. RCOG Press.

Pisarska M, Carson S, Buster J (1998) Ectopic pregnancy. *Lancet* **351**: 1115–20.

Tay JI, Moore J, Walker JJ, Ectopic pregnancy. *BMJ* **320**: 916–19.

Case 31 A breast lump that disappears

Charlotte was a 39-year-old woman with no significant past medical history. She consulted Dr Duffield because she had felt a lump in her left breast the day before. Dr Duffield examined both breasts but could find no abnormality or asymmetry.

What would you do now?

Dr Duffield advised Charlotte that she could find no abnormality but to return if she felt that her left breast had changed or that she could feel a lump.

Two years later Charlotte consulted another general practitioner at the practice with a breast lump. There was a palpable lump and the doctor referred her urgently under the UK NHS 'Two Week Rule' guidance. Charlotte was diagnosed with a left breast cancer and underwent a local excision. The histological diameter of the tumour was 17 mm.

Do you think her claim will succeed?

 Expert comment

Delayed or missed diagnoses of breast cancer remain very common causes of claims against general practitioners and, increasingly, nurse practitioners. The standard required of the general practitioner is very straightforward and the cases normally come down to the question of whether or not the breast examination was competently carried out. Surprisingly, there are still general practitioners, usually of the older generation, who either examine the woman while seated or examine only one breast. The correct examination technique is set out in many textbooks and also in the excellent review article 'Does this patient have breast cancer?' (Barton *et al.*, 1999).

The standard required of UK general practitioners is objectively fairly simple and is set out in the 2005 NICE guidance document: *Referral Guidelines for Suspected Cancer in Adults and Children* and in *Guidelines for the Referral of Patients with Breast Problems* (Austoker & Mansel, 2003).

In a woman aged 30 years and older with a discrete lump that persists after her next period, or presents after menopause, an urgent referral should be made. A woman with asymmetric ('dominant') breast nodularity who is aged under 35 without a family history of breast cancer should be re-examined after an interval and, if the asymmetry has disappeared, she should be reassured.

In practice these cases tend to come down to the question of whether or not the lump should have been detected to competent examination. They are cases in which the question of the cell kinetics of tumours, normally only relevant to specialists commenting on the consequences of any breach of duty (medical causation), become relevant to the question of breach of duty.

What size was the lump likely to be two years earlier? The second question is what size of lump is detectable to competent examination by an average general practitioner?

The standard simplified model of tumour growth is that of exponential (Gompertzian) growth. The first cancerous cell divides and the cells continue to double in number and size once every set period of time. This time is the tumour volume doubling time. Aggressive tumours may double every 10–20 days while more indolent tumours may have doubling times of a year or more. Some awareness of cancer kinetics and the performance characteristics of clinical breast examination (CBE) may inform decisions about how to approach the problem of a patient's subjectively noticed breast asymmetry.

The human body is made up of about 10^{13} cells or about 2^{41} cells. A lethal cancer load is unlikely to contain more than 2^{40} cells. It takes 40 doubling times to reach this extent. A 5 mm diameter cancer has about 2^{27}

Avoiding Errors in General Practice, First Edition. Kevin Barraclough, Jenny du Toit, Jeremy Budd, Joseph E. Raine, Kate Williams and Jonathan Bonser.
© 2013 John Wiley & Sons, Ltd. Published 2013 by John Wiley & Sons, Ltd.

cells and a 1 cm tumour about 2^{30} cells (it takes 3 volume doubling times for the tumour to double in linear diameter).

Breast cancers in women under the age of 50 have doubling times of about 44–147 days with a mean of 80 days. For patients over 50 the mean is 157 days with a range of 121–204 days (Peer *et al.*, 1993). Thus, by the time the tumour is 1 cm in size it has divided about 30 times and death would probably be in another 10 doubling times. A tumour that is 1 cm in diameter will be 2 cm in diameter 3 volume doubling times later. This increase in size may take anything from four months to two years.

How sensitive is clinical breast examination (CBE)?

There are a number of factors that are likely to determine whether a breast lump is clinically palpable. The most important factor is likely to be the size of the lump. Other factors are likely to be:

1. the lump's 'hardness' relative to the surround tissue;
2. the depth on the lump in the breast;
3. the amount of irregularity or nodularity in the surrounding breast;
4. whether the woman is obese or not obese;
5. whether the woman is pre or post menopausal.

One retrospective study described above was carried out on 509 consecutive cases of women diagnosed with breast cancer at a university breast unit (Reintgen *et al.*, 1993). Experienced breast surgeons attempted to palpate the tumour and then the size of the tumour was determined histologically after surgical resection.

The breast surgeons were aware of the mammogram findings at the time of examination. They were therefore aware of the likelihood that the patient had cancer and the site of that cancer.

The results are given in Case Table 31.1.

Another influential study was Oestreicher *et al.* (2002) which looked at a study population of 468 women aged 40 or older who were diagnosed with breast cancer at clinical screening by CBE or were diagnosed within one year of a negative CBE (usually by mammography).

Case Table 31.1 Mammogram results of patient.

Tumour size (mm)	Percentage detectable by CBE
< 5	0
6–10	9
11–15	8
16–20	2

Case Table 31.2 The effect of tumour size on detection rate on CBE.

Characteristic	Women with true positive CBE result, $N = 165$	Women with false negative CBE result, $N = 303$	Row % (sensitivity)
Tumor size at diagnosis			
$\leq$0.5 cm	5	24	17.2%
0.6–1.0 cm	30	107	21.9%
1.1–2.0 cm	81	123	39.7%
$\geq$2.1 cm	42	30	58.3%
p for trend			<0.001

Of the 428 women with breast cancer, 165 were detected at CBE. 303 were not diagnosed at CBE but were subsequently diagnosed by mammography (257) or because of the patient detecting a lump within the next 12 months (46).

Thus the overall sensitivity of CBE for detecting breast cancer was 35% (165/428).

The effect of tumour size on detection rate on CBE is given Case Table 31.2.

The first study suggests that even under optimal conditions (specialist breast surgeons examining and the diagnosis is known) more than 50% of tumours sized 11–15 mm were not detectable. The second, possibly more realistic study suggests that only 40% were detectable at up to 2 cm in size.

These studies suggest that CBE is fairly insensitive at detecting tumours in the 1–2 cm size range. Hence caution and a low threshold for re-examination are probably indicated.

If a lump is detected the management is straightforward. However, if a woman detects a lump and the doctor cannot it may be wise to re-examine the woman in six weeks (and possibly even again in three months). Re-examination is required if there is asymmetry, because of the guidance.

In this case it was unlikely that the tumour would have been detectable to competent clinical examination two years earlier. If the tumour volume doubling time was about 80 days there would have been roughly 9 volume doubling times or 3 linear doubling times. At first examination the tumour would have been 1/8th of its final diameter, or about 2 mm in size and therefore undetectable.

However, an important point was that Dr Duffield recorded her advice that CBE could potentially miss tumours and that if Charlotte felt a change in her breast or detected a lump subsequently she should return.

Legal comment

The question is posed: 'Do you think her [Charlotte's] claim will succeed?' The short answer is no. It seems likely that an oncology expert will conclude that the tumour was only 2 mm in size, when Charlotte consulted with Dr Duffield. This would not have been detectable. Furthermore, Dr Duffield noted good advice for safetynetting. It should, therefore, be possible to defend Dr Duffield's standard of care.

However, Charlotte's own lawyers will probably not even seek an expert opinion. To have a claim of any sort, Charlotte has to show that the alleged breach of duty or failure on the part of Dr Duffield has made a material difference to outcome. Charlotte underwent local excision. This is probably what would have happened if the tumour had been detected earlier. The difference would have been negligible. Therefore, there is no claim.

However, if Charlotte's tumour recurs in future years, she may want to return to her lawyers to see if earlier treatment would have prevented that recurrence and its sequelae. But she will still face the problem that Dr Duffield's care seems to have been appropriate.

Key learning points

Specific to the case

• The standard required of general practitioners when assessing possible breast cancer is very simple. Women over 30 with a discrete lump that persists after the next period need to be referred urgently. A woman with significant breast asymmetry needs to be re examined after the next period and referred if it persists.

• In cases of alleged delay in detecting a breast cancer the question is usually whether a competent general practitioner would have detected the lump

at the earlier examination. A lump will double in linear size in 3 volume doubling times or between about 4 months and 2 years.

• Good quality studies indicate that clinical breast examination is relatively poor at detecting smaller lumps. It is possible that only 40% of lumps in the size range 1.1 cm to 2.0 cm are detectable.

• Consequently, it is wise to have a low threshold for re-examination after an interval and to formulate 'safety netting' advice with suitable cautions about the sensitivity of breast examination and advise immediate return if any change is detected.

General points

• It is always useful, where possible, to know the limitations of the clinical tools – clinical features or tests – that we use and to formulate our 'safety netting' advice according to the degree of uncertainty.

References

Austoker J, Mansel R (2003) *Guidelines for the Referral of Patients with Breast Problems*. NHS Cancer Screening Programmes.

Barton M, Harris R, Fletcher SW (1999) Does this patient have breast cancer? *Journal of American Medical Association* **282**: 1270–81.

Peer PG, van Dijk JA, Hendriks JH, Holland R, Verbeek AL (1993) Age dependent growth rate of breast cancer. *Cancer* **71**: 3547–51.

Reintgen D, Berman C, Cox C, Baekey P, Nicosia S, Greenberg H *et al.* (1993) The anatomy of missed breast cancers. *Surgical Oncology* **2**: 65–75.

Oestreicher N, White E, Lehman CD, Mandelson MT, Porter PL, Taplin SH (2002) Predictors of sensitivity of clinical breast examination (CBE). *Breast Cancer Research and Treatment* **76**: 73–81.

NICE (2005) *NICE Guidance Document: Referral Guidelines for Suspected Cancer in Adults and Children*. CG027.

Case 32 Fever and cough after an ankle fusion

Ethel was 68. At the age of 23 she was knocked off her bicycle by a car and fractured her left ankle. Over recent years her ankle had become increasingly painful. An X-ray confirmed secondary osteoarthritis of the left ankle and an orthopaedic surgeon performed an ankle fusion. Although Ethel had a slight pyrexia she was discharged from hospital four days later in a below knee cast with crutches.

The following day Ethel's husband requested a home visit because he was worried about his wife. She felt feverish and had developed a cough. Dr Macdonald visited at 3 pm. He noted that Ethel had had ankle surgery five days earlier and now had a cough. On examination her temperature was 37.1 °C, although her husband said it had been 38.5 °C earlier in the day. On chest auscultation Dr Macdonald found crackles at the left base. The below-knee plaster did not appear to be too tight and Ethel was able to move her toes. Dr Macdonald prescribed amoxicillin 250 mg tds for a presumed chest infection.

Would you have done anything differently?

Later that evening Ethel's husband went to check on her. She was confused and disorientated. He rang NHS direct who advised him to dial '999'. When the ambulance arrived at 10 pm Ethel had a temperature of 39.5 °C. Her pulse was 140/min, BP 85/50 and an oxygen saturation of 86%. She was taken to hospital.

The admitting doctor recorded a 2-day history of fever and breathlessness and a cough that day. There was no headache or photophobia. Findings on examination were temperature 40, pulse rate 160, BP 100/60, respiratory rate 30/min, generalized erythema but peripheral cyanosis and scattered crackles in the chest. A

diagnosis of suspected septicaemia was made and Ethel was admitted to the ICU. She developed renal failure and despite intensive treatment she died. A post-mortem showed changes in keeping with septic shock. A toxin producing Staphlococcus aureus was isolated from the lungs and left ankle.

It was alleged that Dr Macdonald's assessment was inadequate and that had he adequately assessed Ethel he would have admitted her to hospital.

Do you think the claim will succeed?

 ## Expert comment

Early discharge of patients post-operatively is occurring more frequently and general practitioners need to be able to assess problems that arise. Mild degrees of fever are usually caused by infection but can also be caused by venous thrombosis. Many minor post operative infections can be treated in the community with oral antibiotics and do not require readmission. Thus, most competent general practitioners would routinely treat patients at home with superficial wound infections, minor degrees of cellulitis, bronchitis, pneumonia (if the patient is low risk) or a urinary tract infection.

Indications for admission would usually be:
- a clinical suspicion of septicaemia;
- pneumonia with 'high-risk' features as defined in the British Thoracic Society Guidelines (respiratory rate over 30, low blood pressure, confusion, co-morbidity);
- a clinical suspicion of DVT;
- a wound abscess that is likely to need surgical drainage;
- clinical suspicion of an occult abscess;
- a pyrexia in which the cause is uncertain.

Avoiding Errors in General Practice, First Edition. Kevin Barraclough, Jenny du Toit, Jeremy Budd, Joseph E. Raine, Kate Williams and Jonathan Bonser.
© 2013 John Wiley & Sons, Ltd. Published 2013 by John Wiley & Sons, Ltd.

Septicaemia would be suspected if a patient has any of the following features:
- a high fever (often taken as being over 38.5 C°);
- systemic symptoms of rigors or sweats;
- confusion;
- a petechial rash;
- features of septic shock: low blood pressure (systolic < 100 mmHg), fast heart rate (over 100 at rest), low urine output, mottled skin colour, cold peripheries;
- headache in a febrile patient with any of the above features would lead a general practitioner to consider the possibility of meningitis with septicaemia.

Therefore when assessing the recent onset of fever in a post-operative patient a general practitioner should enquire about the following:
- symptoms that may give an indication of a focus of infection – symptoms of pneumonia or bronchitis, symptoms of a urinary tract infection, wound pain or headache;
- symptoms that may suggest septicaemia: rigors, sweats, confusion, headaches, nausea, vomiting or diarrhoea.

In 2006 Thompson et al. (Thompson et al., 2006) described more subtle and earlier clinical features of meningococcal septicaemia in children and young adults. They identified three features in particular: cold hands and feet; leg pain; and abnormal skin colour (pallor or mottling).

The temperature pulse and blood pressure should always be measured to differentiate minor infection from septicaemia. The general practitioner should also examine the wound for signs of infection, listen to the chest, recording the respiratory rate if a chest infection is suspected, and dipstick the urine if there are symptoms of a urinary tract infection or the cause of the pyrexia is unclear. Capillary refill time should be assessed, although the evidence for its usefulness is relatively poor (Lewin & Maconochie, 2008). It is also important in the post-operative patient to check the legs for signs of a DVT.

In this case Dr MacDonald's entry in the notes was rather brief. He does not appear to have ascertained if the cough was productive or associated with breathless or chest pain. There is no record to suggest that he enquired about other possible causes of a post-operative pyrexia. Although he recorded the temperature he failed to record Ethel's pulse rate and blood pressure. He did look at Ethel's left leg but gives no indication that he considered the possibility of a DVT.

If the patients pulse and blood pressure had been normal, Dr MacDonald's presumptive diagnosis of a chest infection would be reasonable. Ethel had had a raised temperature earlier in the day and had a cough and chest signs (Lewin & Maconochie, 2008). However the dose of antibiotic he prescribed was inadequate. The Health Protection Agency recommend amoxicillin 500–1000 mg tds for an adult with a community acquired pneumonia.

If Ethel had had a tachycardia (PR > 100 at rest) or hypotension (systolic blood pressure < 100–110) then Dr Donald should have suspected more serious sepsis and admitted her.

It may be that Ethel was not particularly unwell when she was seen and that her condition deteriorated rapidly over the course of the evening. In this circumstance the diagnosis of septicaemia would have been understandably missed.

The difficulty with the case for Dr Donald's defence is that, because the pulse and blood pressure have not been recorded, it remains uncertain whether Ethel had clinical features of septicaemia at the time of his assessment. Dr Donald's poor note-keeping may be taken by the Court to indicate poor practice. In addition Dr MacDonald did not record providing any safety netting advice.

 Legal comment

We do not know whether Ethel looked particularly unwell. But this could simply reflect the poor standard of Dr Donald's note-keeping. It will be difficult for him to prove just how well she was. This in itself will make it difficult to defend the standard of care provided to Ethel. But it may be that on her husband's own evidence Ethel's condition would not have warranted immediate admission. The question would then be whether Dr Donald's safety-netting was good enough.

At the very most, Ethel would have been admitted to hospital six or seven hours earlier than she was. An expert in infectious diseases will be asked to give his opinion on whether earlier admission would have saved her life.

The case may be worth £50 000, depending on Ethel's role in the marriage. The case is not straightforward. The parties will probably negotiate a settlement at a discount on the full valuation.

Key learning points

Specific to the case
• It is essential to bear in mind a full differential diagnosis when assessing a patient with postoperative pyrexia.
• Temperature pulse and blood pressure should always be measured and recorded to differentiate minor postoperative infection from septicaemia.

General points
• This case highlights the need for a good consultation note.

References

British Thoracic Society (2001) Guidelines for the management of community acquired pneumonia in adults. *Thorax* **56**:1iv-64.

Lewin J, Maconochie I (2008) Capillary refill time in adults. *Emergency Medicine Journal* **25**: 325–6.

Metlay JP, Kapoor WN, Fine MJ (1997) Does this patient have community-acquired pneumonia? Diagnosing pneumonia by history and physical examination. *JAMA* **278**: 1440–5.

Thompson MJ, Ninis N, Perera R, Mayon-White R, Phillips C, Bailey L *et al.* (2006) Clinical recognition of meningococcal disease in children and adolescents. *The Lancet* **367**: 397–403.

Case 33 Urinary problem in a welder

Reg was a 60-year-old self-employed welder when he consulted Dr Oakley. He had noted that he had had rather poor urinary stream and hesitancy for a year or so. A programme he had seen on the TV caused him to think that he needed to be checked out for prostate cancer.

Dr Oakley checked Reg's International Prostate Symptom Score and it was 11/35. This suggested symptoms of prostatism of moderate severity. Digital rectal examination showed a large, firm but benign feeling prostate with a central sulcus. A week later Reg had a PSA which was 7.2 ng/ml.

What would you do now?

Reg returned to see Dr Oakley. Reg was very concerned that his PSA was raised. Dr Oakley explained that it was a rather poor test and that many male doctors may not have wanted to have a PSA test done on themselves because it was such a poor test.

They agreed that Reg would have the test repeated in 3 months. At that stage the PSA was 8.1 ng/dl. After discussion they agreed that Reg would have it repeated again in 6 months. Unfortunately Reg forgot to return for the test and it was eventually repeated 22 months later. At this stage the PSA was found to be 16 ng/dl. Dr Oakley referred Reg. He was found to have a locally invasive prostate cancer that had infiltrated the seminal vesicles and he was not suitable for radical prostatectomy.

Reg was angry that he had not been referred initially, when his PSA was only 7.2. He had been told that if he had been referred at that stage he could have had curative surgery. He brought a claim against Dr Oakley.

Do you think his claim will succeed?

 Expert comment

This case illustrates a number of difficult areas for general practitioners with regard to PSA tests, adherence to guidelines and the notion of informed consent.

Many general practitioners would probably not have a PSA done on themselves because of the low specificity of the test and the fact that localized prostate can probably be detected in 15% to 30% of 50 year olds (Selley *et al.*, 1997). Yet only 3% of the male population die of prostate cancer and the median age of death for the condition is 80. The difficulty, of course, is knowing who should be left alone and who may come to harm. As the 2002 NHS Prostate Cancer Risk Management Program puts it:

> Prostate cancer is not a single disease entity but more a spectrum of diseases ranging from very aggressive to slow growing tumours, which may not cause any symptoms or shorten life. Many men with less aggressive disease tend to die *with* rather than *of* their cancer, but it is not always possible to tell at diagnosis which tumours are aggressive and which are slow growing.

An additional difficulty is that 10% of PSAs done in men aged 50 to 60 will be 'raised' (Wilt & Thompson, 2006).

Despite this the July 2000 Department of Health (DOH) guidelines for Referral of patients with Suspected Cancer advised urgent referral of all men with an elevated age specific PSA in men with a ten year life expectancy. This comprises 10% of the male population between the age of 50 and 60. The 2005 NICE version of the referral guidelines modified the situation slightly, but also slightly complicated the issue by stating:

> If there is doubt about whether to refer an asymptomatic male with a borderline level of PSA, the PSA test should be repeated after an interval of 1 to 3 months. If the second test indicates that the PSA level is rising, the patient should be referred urgently.

Dr Oakley had attended a lecture by his local urologist who had pointed out the difficulties with the DOH guidance and who had expressed personal views about who should and should not be referred urgently. The

Avoiding Errors in General Practice, First Edition. Kevin Barraclough, Jenny du Toit, Jeremy Budd, Joseph E. Raine, Kate Williams and Jonathan Bonser.

urologist pointed out that the department were at that time swamped with such referrals and were struggling to see other patients within a reasonable time.

This case illustrates the difficulty for general practitioners when following over-inclusive guidance would swamp local services (and generate large amounts of anxiety), but failure to follow the guidelines may lead to censure. A similar example of such guidance is the '7 point' criteria for urgent referral of pigmented lesions as possible malignant melanomas. The specificity of the rules is so low that general practitioners following the letter of the guidance would refer 60% of pigmented lesions urgently.

However, in this case there were a number of problems. Dr Oakley was not aware that a rising PSA at > 0.75 ng/ml per year (in the US 0.35 ng/ml/yr is taken as significant) probably has a greater predictive value for clinically significant prostate cancer than a single raised reading. He did not communicate this to Reg because he did not know it.

Reg argued that he had not been put in a position to make the decision as to whether he wished to be referred or not because Dr Oakley had not given him the information in the NHS Prostate Cancer Risk Management Program. Reg stated that he had been unaware of the significance of the rising PSA and Dr Oakley had imposed his own views about PSAs on Reg and had not followed national guidelines. Reg had been advised that his chance of having biopsy proven prostate cancer on the first occasion was about 45% and of having 'high-grade cancer' was about 10%.

It would certainly not be possible to defend the allegation of breach of duty at the time of the second PSA result because Dr Oakley had not realized the significance of a rising PSA and had not given Reg sufficient information to allow him to make his own decision about referral. However, the guidance as it stands does put general practitioners in a difficult position.

 Legal comment

Dr Oakley should have referred Reg after the second PSA. This is a clear breach of duty. Whether Reg will succeed in his claim will depend on the causation evidence of a urologist or an oncologist. Causation in cancer cases is not straightforward. It is generally based on five- or ten-year survival rates and how these change from the time when diagnosis should have been made until it was actually made.

That said, it appears likely that Reg will be able to show that he could have been cured, if Dr Oakley had referred him. The calculation of the damages will not be a straightforward affair, either. Keeping it simple, Reg could be compensated for loss of life expectancy during his lifetime or if he is married, his wife could benefit from damages after his death.

 Key learning points

Specific to the case
- A rising PSA (greater than 0.75 ng/ml) probably has a greater predictive value for identifying progressive prostate cancer than a single test result.
- It is helpful to make use of the printed material produced by the NHS Prostate Cancer Risk Management Program to help make decisions about PSA tests.

General points
- Over inclusive referral guidelines can put general practitioners in a vulnerable position if negligence is alleged and they did not adhere to the guidelines.
- If a patient is going to give 'informed dissent', deciding not to be referred or investigated, it is only a defence if the patient was given all information that a reasonable person would consider pertinent to making the decision.

References

Selley S, Donovan J, Faulkner A, Coast J, Gillatt D (1997) Diagnosis, management and screening of early localized prostate cancer. *Health Technol Assess* **1**(2).

Wilt T, Thompson I (2006) Clinically localized prostate cancer. *BMJ* **333**: 1102–6.

Case 34 A hypertensive 38-year-old woman

Diana had her second child at the age of 32. Her blood pressure was first noted to be slightly high towards the end of this pregnancy. At the postnatal check her blood pressure was 140/90 mmHg. Over the subsequent two years her blood pressure was measured on a few occasions. The readings showed systolic pressures of 150–160 mmHg and diastolic pressures of 90–100. Diana's creatinine and cholesterol were normal.

Dr Williams decided to treat her with atenolol.

What would you do now?

During the next four years, follow-up was rather intermittent and Diana's compliance with medication somewhat erratic. Blood pressure readings ranged between 160–180 mmHg and 90–105 mmHg.

In 2009, at the age of 38, Diana had a sudden onset of severe headache and collapsed at home. She was admitted to hospital and found to have had a right middle cerebral artery haemorrhage. Diana had a craniotomy and evacuation of the cerebral haematoma. Unfortunately she only made a partial recovery and was left with a severe left hemiparesis. She is only able to walk up to 100 yards with a stick and requires a wheelchair for longer distances. Subsequent investigation revealed that her hypertension was secondary to polycystic kidneys.

It was alleged that Dr Williams should have investigated Diana to determine if there was a secondary cause for her hypertension in view of her young age. It was alleged that if she had been investigated she would have been found to have polycystic kidneys and that this would have prompted referral to a nephrologist. This would have resulted in earlier and better control of her hypertension. In addition it was alleged that Diana's hypertension was inadequately treated.

 ### Expert comment

The Health Survey for England 2009 showed that 32 % of men and 27% of women over the age of 35 have a BP

of 140/90 or more or are on treatment for hypertension (NHS, 2009). At least 95% of cases are 'primary', or 'essential hypertension'. Secondary cause of hypertension should be considered in those who are aged 35 or less, in patients with difficult to control hypertension, and in those who have features of an underlying cause.

At the time of this case the British Hypertension Society advised that hypertension should be diagnosed if there were three readings of a blood pressure ≥ 160/100 (Williams *et al.*, 2004). If the blood pressure was between 140/90 and 160/100 the patient's cardiovascular risk should be assessed and the patient treated if this was greater than 20% in 10 years.

These guidelines have been superseded by those published in August 2011 by NICE. In this case it was not clear on what basis the diagnosis of hypertension was made. The choice of antihypertensive medication was appropriate because Diana was of child-bearing age. Dr Williams could have chosen an ACEI in view of her age but would have had to warn her about the need to discontinue the medication should she become pregnant. The latest guidance is that ACE inhibitors, angiotensin receptor blockers and chlorothiazide are teratogenic and should not be used in pregnancy. The limited evidence available does not show an increase in congenital abnormalities with any other antihypertensive treatment (NICE, 2011).

The most problematic issue is that Dr Williams does not seem to have appreciated the need to investigate Diana. Had he done so, the diagnosis of polycystic kidney disease (PKD) would have been made four or five years before Diana had the subarachnoid haemorrhage.

Autosomal dominant PKD is an inherited condition that will affect 50% of the children of a parent who is affected. It is one of the commoner of the inherited diseases and affects between 1 in 400 and 1 in 1000 individuals (Gabow, 1993). Many general practitioners will have one or more patients with the condition.

The condition is usually diagnosed after a renal ultrasound shows multiple cysts in both kidneys. An

---

Avoiding Errors in General Practice, First Edition. Kevin Barraclough, Jenny du Toit, Jeremy Budd, Joseph E. Raine, Kate Williams and Jonathan Bonser.

ultrasound may be requested for several reasons: for the investigation of loin pain (which occurs with PKD), because a relative has the condition, for the investigation of asymptomatic haematuria or to investigate causes of secondary hypertension (Gabow, 1993).

The commonest complication of PKD is the development of hypertension. 60% of adults develop hypertension before they begin to lose any measurable degree of renal function (Gabow, 1993). Cerebral 'Berry aneurysms' are also associated with PKD. The frequency with which berry aneurysms are found in patients with PKD is quoted as anything between 0% and 40%. Three studies which together screened a total of 273 patients with PKD for asymptomatic berry aneurysms found aneurysms in 13 patients (a prevalence of 5%) (Gabow, 1993).

Treatment of hypertension reduces the risk of stroke and heart disease in all patients (whether they have PKD or not). The evidence is that treatment of mild to moderate hypertension (blood pressures of 140 to 180 mmHg systolic and 90 to 110 mmHg diastolic) in patients with 'essential hypertension' (as opposed to those with hypertension secondary to PKD) reduces the risk of stroke by between 30% and 43% (MRC, 1985; Wood *et al.*, 1998). The percentage reduction is likely to be greater for haemorrhagic strokes. However, to 'prove' causation in civil litigation the risk of stroke would have to be reduced by more than 50% (such that the stroke would be more likely than not to have been prevented). Causation experts would be likely to argue this issue in this case.

A further issue, with regard to both breach of duty and causation, is that it can be difficult to adequately treat hypertension. A *BMJ* review in 2004 commented that, with the introduction of newer stringent targets, blood pressure was controlled adequately in only a third of patients (Campbell & Murchie, 2004).

A study among UK general practitioners found widespread scepticism about the evidence base, desirability and achievability of tighter blood pressure target levels (Heneghan *et al.*, 2007). In addition up to 40% of patients treated for hypertension fail to take their medication as prescribed (Vrijens *et al.*, 2008).

However, realistically, breach of duty could not be defended.

Even in the light of the difficulties outlined above the doctors in the practice did not manage Diana's blood pressure adequately. Diana's blood pressure was checked infrequently and was always above a target level of 140/85. Usual practice would have been for her to have had her blood pressure taken every 6 months once it was adequately controlled.

Furthermore, Diana should have been investigated for secondary causes of hypertension because she was very young to have essential hypertension.

Had the diagnosis of PKD had been made earlier Diana should have been referred to a nephrologist. In these circumstances the blood pressure may well have been more aggressively managed with a view to slowing the deterioration of renal function. The target level for blood pressure would have been 130/80. In addition Diana might have been more motivated to take her medication regularly.

 Legal comment

It will prove difficult to defend Dr Williams's standard of care. At the end of the day, the causation experts are likely to conclude that with appropriate treatment, Diana would not have suffered her stroke. However, causation is not straightforward. There are a number of arguments (surrounding the difficulties in controlling hypertension) that Dr Williams's lawyers will be able to use to negotiate a discounted settlement.

The level of damages will depend largely on how badly Diana's disability affects her life. Damages could easily be in the high hundreds of thousands of pounds.

 Key learning points

Specific to the case
- Although secondary causes of hypertension are uncommon they should always be considered in young patients.

General points
- A system for the follow-up of chronic disease and the use of templates helps not only to assist adequate management but also enables this to be demonstrated.

References

Campbell NC, Murchie P (2004) Treating hypertension with guidelines in general practice. *BMJ* **329**: 523–4.

Gabow PA (1993) Autosomal dominant polycystic kidney disease. *N Engl J Med* **329**: 332–42.

Heneghan C, Perera R, Mant D, Glasziou P (2007) Hypertension guideline recommendations in general practice: awareness, agreement, adoption and adherence. *British Journal of General Practice* **57**: 948–52.

Medical Research Council (1985) Treatment of mild hypertension: principal results. *BMJ* **291**: 97–104.

NHS (2009) Health Survey for England. National Health Service.

NICE (2011) NICE Guidance on hypertension in pregnancy.

Vrijens B, Vincze G, Kristano P, Urquhart J, Burnier M (2008) Adherence to prescribing antihypertensive drug treatments: longtitudinal study of electronically compiled dosing histories. *BMJ* **336**: 1114–17.

Williams B, Poulter NR, Brown MJ, Davis M, McInnes GT, Potter JF, Sever PS, McG Thom S (2004) British Hypertension Society Guidelines for the hypertension management 2004 (SHS-IV). *BMJ* **328**: 634–40.

Wood D, Durrington P, Poulter N, *et al.* (1998) Joint British recommendations on prevention of coronary heart disease in clinical practice. *Heart* **80**: S1–29.

Case 35 A swollen lip in a 56-year-old man

James was a 56-year-old man. He was hypertensive with a strong family history of coronary disease. He was taking aspirin, a statin, a beta blocker and had recently started an ACE inhibitor for blood pressure control. He consulted Dr Patten after Monday morning surgery with a history that, on the Sunday evening his lip had become very swollen when he drank coke with his children in a fast food restaurant. His lip had reverted to normal size after a few hours.

What would you do now?

Dr Patten considered that it was most likely an allergic reason to the coke and advised him to avoid the drink in future. Three weeks later James consulted a colleague with a swollen itchy scrotum. The general practitioner considered it was probably an allergic reaction to washing powder.

What would be your differential diagnosis and how would you discriminate between them?

A month later James consulted Dr Patten again. He had had a recurrence of a rather severe back pain after lifting his son's drum set into the car. He was taking paracetamol but the pain was not controlled. Dr Patten prescribed diclofenac and co-codamol.

The next day, after taking the diclofenac, James began to experience shortness of breath and his face and tongue started to swell. His wife called an ambulance but James suffered a respiratory arrest from which he was resuscitated. In hospital he was diagnosed with anaphylaxis caused by taking diclofenac and possibly contributed to by being on an ACE inhibitor.

He brought a claim against Dr Patten and his colleague alleging that they should have recognized that the swelling of his lip and scrotum were suggestive of angio-oedema and that the ACE inhibitor should have

been stopped. It was alleged that James had some degree of memory impairment from his hypoxic episode.

Do you think his claim will succeed?

 Expert comment

The vast majority of claims against general practitioners are for failure to diagnose or delay in diagnosis or referral. However, a proportion are about negligent prescribing, failure to adequately monitor drug therapy (for example lithium, phenytoin, amiodarone or methotrexate) or failure to recognize significant side effects.

In this case it was not clear that Dr Patten recognized that the episode described by James was due to angio-oedema. The rapid swelling of the lip followed by relatively rapid resolution was typical of the condition. Scrotal swelling is also common.

Urticaria, angio-oedema and anaphylaxis are all related conditions. Urticaria and angio-oedema both cause swelling of tissues because the small blood vessels (capillaries) abruptly leak fluid into the tissues. With urticaria the leakage occurs into the superficial tissues of the skin. With angio-oedema the same process occurs with deeper tissues – the dermis (lying below the superficial skin) and mucosal tissues that line the mouth, tongue and airways. The main concern, of course, is the possibility of life-threatening anaphylaxis or airway obstruction. Urticaria is very common in primary care. Angio-oedema is regularly seen but is less common than urticaria. Anaphylaxis is thankfully rare and occurs approximately in 1 person in 10 000 per year and most general practitioners will only encounter it a few times in their clinical career (Ewsan, 1998).

In this case Dr Patten should really have been aware that one of the problems with ACE inhibitors is an increased risk of angio-oedema.

Avoiding Errors in General Practice, First Edition. Kevin Barraclough, Jenny du Toit, Jeremy Budd, Joseph E. Raine, Kate Williams and Jonathan Bonser.
© 2013 John Wiley & Sons, Ltd. Published 2013 by John Wiley & Sons, Ltd.

A reasonable general practitioner should take a very careful history with angio-oedema, because of the potential seriousness of the condition for the future (even if the patient is not currently unwell). The history should include unusual exposures to possible allergens and a drug history.

Drugs, especially penicillins and aspirin, are a common cause of urticaria, angio-oedema and anaphylaxis. In addition regular prescription medication should be checked. Angiotensin Converting Enzyme Inhibitors (ACE inhibitors) are well-recognized causes of urticaria and angio-oedema. In the British National Formulary (BNF) angio-oedema is listed prominently as one of the commoner side effects of ACE inhibitors.

It is not possible for general practitioners to have an encyclopaedic knowledge of the side effects of all drugs. However, many symptoms are caused by (and often unrecognized as) drug side effects. A general practitioner should have a very low threshold for consulting reference texts such as the BNF.

 Legal comment

Starting at the question of damages, if James can prove his case, then he will be compensated for the collapse he experienced. He will also receive damages for his memory impairment, if a neurologist concludes that this was probably due to hypoxia during the episode.

The respiratory arrest was undoubtedly caused by the angio-oedema, so the question that needs to be addressed is: should the general practitioners have diagnosed the condition and stopped the prescription of the ACE inhibitor? The expert opinion above suggests that although Dr Patten and his colleague may not be criticized for failing to realize that James was suffering from angio-oedema, they should have consulted the BNF and this would have led to the diagnosis and revealed the ACE inhibitor as the cause of the condition. On this analysis, the claim will have to be settled.

The value of the claim is difficult to assess without precise information over the level of memory impairment and how it affects James's life and in particular his employment. The claim could be worth tens of thousands or several hundred thousand pounds.

 Key learning points

Specific to the case
- A patient with a history suggestive of angio-oedema will often be perfectly well at the time of assessment. Nevertheless, a very careful history is necessary and, in particular, a careful scrutiny of drug therapy.
- ACE inhibitors are commonly prescribed drugs and are common causes of angio-oedema. Other drugs such as penicillins, aspirin and other NSAIDs are also common precipitants.

General points
- It is not possible for general practitioners to have an encyclopaedic knowledge of the side effects of all drugs. However, a general practitioner should have a very low threshold for consulting reference texts such as the BNF.

Reference

Ewan PW (1998) ABC of allergies: Anaphylaxis. *BMJ* **316**: 1442–5.

Case 36 A woman with fatigue and weight gain

Christina consulted Dr Francis in January 2008. She was worried because she felt tired all the time and had put on weight. A friend who had similar symptoms had been treated with thyroxine for an under-active thyroid and Christina wondered if she might have the same problem. Christina had always been a little over weight and had sought medical advice regarding this before. She did not have any other features to suggest hypothyroidism. She was not taking any medication but had a Mirena for contraception. Her grandmother had had some sort of thyroid problem.

Dr Francis performed a blood test to check the FBC and TSH. The results were normal. The TSH was 5.0 mmol/l.

Christina returned in February to discuss the results. Despite the normal TSH she wanted to try thyroid replacement.

What would you do now?

Dr Francis repeated the TSH and checked for TPO antibodies. Again the TSH was normal at 4.5 mU/l. The TPO antibody tire was 5 IU/l (normal). A few years earlier Dr Francis had looked after a similar patient who had seen a private endocrinologist and been treated with thyroxine. He therefore decided to treat Christina despite the normal thyroid function tests. He prescribed thyroxine 25 micrograms daily. The dose was gradually increased to 100 micrograms daily over the following six months. TSH measurements in April, June and August were 1.0 mU/l, 0.2 mU/l and 0.1 mU/l respectively. On the last occasion the free T4 was 25.1 pmol/l (just over the normal range).

Would you have done the same?

In November Christina came to see another partner at the practice complaining of palpitations and breathlessness. On examination she was in atrial fibrillation. This was attributed to the thyroxine that she was taking.

It was alleged that Dr Francis was negligent because no competent doctor would diagnose hypothyroidism with normal blood tests.

 Expert comment

Hypothyroidism is relatively common. The annual incidence is 3.5 per 1000 women and 0.6 per 1000 men (Vaidya & Pearce, 2008). The symptoms of hypothyroidism (such as fatigue, weight gain or feeling cold) are very nonspecific. Many people without thyroid disease experience these symptoms and seek medical advice. There is good evidence that patients with symptoms suggestive of hypothyroidism but with normal thyroid function do not benefit, either physically or psychologically, from treatment with thyroxine (Pollock *et al.*, 2001)

To answer uncertainties about the use of thyroid tests the Association for Clinical Biochemistry, the British Thyroid Association and the British Thyroid Foundation produced evidence-based guidelines in June 2006.

Thyroxine has been used, particularly in non-NHS clinics, to treat nonthyroid disease such as obesity, chronic fatigue, infertility, menstrual irregularity and short stature (Roti *et al.*, 1993) This has been a cause for concern within the medical community.

In response to these concerns the Royal College of Physicians and the British Thyroid Association produced a policy statement to clarify preexisting guidance in 2008 (RCP/BTA, 2008). This policy statement and the UK Guidelines for the Use of Thyroid Function Tests produced by the Association for Clinical Biochemistry and the British Thyroid Association in July 2006

Avoiding Errors in General Practice, First Edition. Kevin Barraclough, Jenny du Toit, Jeremy Budd, Joseph E. Raine, Kate Williams and Jonathan Bonser.
© 2013 John Wiley & Sons, Ltd. Published 2013 by John Wiley & Sons, Ltd.

(ACB/BTA, 2006) give the following guidance for the diagnosis of primary hypothyroidism:

- A TSH >10 and a Free T4 below the reference range are required for the diagnosis of primary hypothyroidism.
- A TSH within the normal range excludes primary hypothyroidism (as long as the patient is not taking any medication known to affect the TSH).
- Patients with a normal TSH should not be diagnosed with hypothyroidism and should not be treated with thyroxine.

The diagnosis of hypothyroidism must be made on the basis of biochemical tests and not on the basis of clinical symptoms alone.

The inappropriate use of thyroxine is harmful.

- It exposes patients to possible or, as in this case, actual harm. Hyperthyroidism is known to be associated with atrial fibrillation.
- A nonthyroid cause of the symptoms may be missed.

In this case Dr Francis should not have diagnosed hypothyroidism or given Christina thyroxine. If Dr Francis had been concerned that Christina had secondary hypothyroidism she would have had other symptoms to suggest pituitary failure such as headache, visual field disturbance, cranial nerve palsies (II, IV or VI) or features of other endocrine deficiencies such as amenorrhoea, loss of libido etc. Specialist referral would have been required. In addition he did not explore other possible causes for the patient's symptoms such as mental health issues or diabetes.

 Legal comment

Dr Francis's MDO will have to settle this claim. It is clearly indefensible. However, damages will be low, as there will be no long term sequelae from the treatment.

Dr Francis may try to argue that he was following the treatment given by a private endocrinologist in a previous patient. Putting it bluntly, this will not wash. He should assess each patient on his or her condition and in an appropriate manner. If such thinking was communicated to Christina, it may provoke a complaint to the GMC, calling into question Dr Francis's fitness to practise.

 Key learning points

Specific to the case
- The diagnosis of hypothyroidism must be made on the basis of biochemical tests and not on the basis of clinical symptoms alone.
- Thyroxine should only be prescribed if a patient has proven hypothyroidism

General points
- Usually it is entirely reasonable for a general practitioner to rely on the advice of a specialist. This will generally provide a complete defence unless it can be shown that a competent general practitioner would have been aware that the advice received was unsafe.

References

ACB/BTA (2006) UK Guidelines for the Use of Thyroid Function Tests. The Association for Clinical Biochemistry and the British Thyroid Association. July 2006 (http://www.british-thyroid-association.org/Guidelines/)

Pollock MA., Sturrock A, Marshall K, Davidson KM, Kelly CJG, McMahon AD, McLaren EH (2001) Thyroxine treatment in patients with symptoms of hypothyroidism but thyroid function tests within the reference range: randomised double blind placebo controlled crossover trial. *BMJ* **323** : 891 doi: 10.1136/bmj.323.7318.891 (published 20 October 2001).

RCP/BTA (2008) The Diagnosis and Management of Primary Hypothyroidism: A statement made on behalf of The Royal College of Physicians in particular its Patient and Carer Network and the Joint Specialty Committee for Endocrinology & Diabetes.

Roti E, Minelli R, Gardini E, Braverman LE (1993) The use and misuse of thyroid hormone. *Endocrine Reviews* **14**: 401–23; doi:10.1210/edrv-14-4-401

Vaidya B, Pearce SHS (2008) Management of hypothyroidism in adults. *BMJ* **337**: a801.

Case 37 A woman told off for ignoring her friends

Jayne was aged 46 when she initially consulted Dr Saad. She had been to the optician the day before because she felt her vision had deteriorated. She had been told off on a few occasions by friends who said that she had ignored them. She had not noticed, or not seen them, as they walked past in the street. The optician had suggested that she see her general practitioner and get referred to hospital.

What would you do now?

Dr Saad measured Jayne's visual acuities. They were normal. Her fundi also appeared normal. Dr Saad was familiar with the optician. The optician was an anxious professional who often sent patients to Dr Saad. Dr Saad reassured Jayne that he could find nothing particular wrong and that referral to hospital did not seem necessary. He suggested review if the problem got worse.

What would be your differential diagnosis and how would you discriminate between them? Would you have done anything else?

Two days later the letter arrived from the optician. An automated field test had showed black squares in the upper outer quadrant of the right eye field and a lesser number of black squares in the right field of the left eye. Dr Saad was not familiar with the printout from the test but the optician suggested non-urgent referral to hospital. Dr Saad decided to refer Jayne for an ophthalmology opinion under the Choose and Book system.

Six months later Jayne consulted Dr Fowler at the practice. She had been experiencing daily headaches for several weeks. They were dull, tended to be worse in the morning and were largely gone by lunchtime. She had also noticed that she seemed to be a bit clumsy when she had the headaches and had been bumping into things.

Dr Fowler did not notice the ophthalmology referral 6 months earlier. It appeared subsequently that Jayne had not known what the Choose and Book letter she was sent was about, and she had taken no action. Jayne's blood pressure and fundi were normal but Dr Fowler thought that Jayne was not seeing out of the lateral field of her right eye. He questioned Jayne about flashing lights (she had had none) deliberated about whether to refer her to neurology or ophthalmology and decided on the latter. He also started her on low-dose pizotifen.

Unfortunately, before she was seen in the ophthalmology clinic Jayne had a fit while driving and crashed. She was unhurt but the driver of the other car was seriously injured. On examination in it was noted that Jayne had a significant visual sensory inattention in the entire right visual field and a largely homonymous field loss extending to about one quarter of her right visual field.

Investigations revealed that Jayne had a large left occipital glioma. The driver of the other car brought an action against Jayne, and Jayne's insurance company brought an action against Dr Saad and Dr Fowler on Jayne's behalf.

Do you think the claim will succeed?

 Expert comment

Cases in which a communication between medical professionals goes astray, or is not acted upon, are common. The communication from the physiotherapist or optician fails to reach the general practitioner, or the general practitioner fails to act upon it. It is also important to recognize that colleagues, such as opticians, physiotherapists, osteopaths etc., do have a great deal of experience in their respective areas and that their findings of something being out of the ordinary or abnormal should be taken seriously.

Avoiding Errors in General Practice, First Edition. Kevin Barraclough, Jenny du Toit, Jeremy Budd, Joseph E. Raine, Kate Williams and Jonathan Bonser.
© 2013 John Wiley & Sons, Ltd. Published 2013 by John Wiley & Sons, Ltd.

In this case there were a number of communication breakdowns. The letter from the optician did not reach Dr Saad until after he had seen Jayne. He then did not communicate his decision to refer her to Jayne herself. Dr Fowler failed to read back in the notes and notice Dr Saad's consultation and the subsequent referral. When significant medical errors occur there is often a concatenation of minor errors that lead to, and contribute to it.

Assessing visual field to confrontation is not a particularly easy skill for a general practitioner and it does require significant care. Ideally each eye should be examined separately with a small object (preferably red – traditionally a hat pin but a red biro top will do!) and then fields should be checked more grossly (wiggling index fingers) with both eyes open. As with many neurological examination skills, general practitioners do not frequently use them and quite often cease to practise them at all. The sad thing with this is that these are proven and useful examination techniques, they cost nothing, and if they are not used, the skill atrophies.

It is also important to recognize the limitations of examination findings and the performance characteristics of tests. A unilateral sensory inattention (stimulus detected on one side when unopposed but extinguished with bilateral stimuli) is quite a difficult sign, but an automated visual field test is very sensitive at detecting field loss. Dr Saad admitted that he was not really familiar with the test or the meaning of the printout he was sent.

Dr Saad should really have sought clarification from the optician, an online textbook or a specialist if he was uncertain about the significance of the field test. The decision to refer Jayne should really have been communicated personally to her. It was predictable that she might be unsure about the 'Choose and Book' letter and not ring to make the necessary appointment.

Dr Fowler should really have looked back at the earlier notes and correspondence. As compared to hospital practice, general practice is characterized by 10-minute consultations about diffuse and multiple matters but the general practitioners, individually or (more commonly now) collectively, build up a large amount of information about a patient over the previous year or years. It is essential to use this resource if the 10-minute consultation is going to be more than a snapshot glimpse of the patient.

Many negligence cases hang on the question of whether the general practitioner should have glanced at the previous notes (usually they should have glanced at a few) or the summary of the past medical history and current drug therapy (almost invariably they should have done so).

The difference between homonymous binocular visual symptoms and uniocular symptoms is an important one. For example right visual field flashing lights are usually occipital in origin and are probably migraine. Flashing lights in the one eye are usually retinal in origin and generally indicate traction due to a posterior vitreous detachment or retinal tear. These are important distinctions and they occur frequently in patients presenting with visual symptoms.

Headaches in isolation are the presenting feature of cerebral tumours in only 2–16% of primary cerebral tumours, and are the cause of headaches in only about 0.1% of all consultations about headache (Hamilton & Kernick, 2007). Most cerebral tumours present with a fit. About 1.2% of patients in general practice with a first fit have a tumour as the cause (Hamilton & Kernick, 2007). Case control studies have not shown that headache on waking is a particularly useful clinical feature to predict a cerebral tumour.

It would not be possible to defend breach of duty on behalf of Dr Saad. A competent general practitioner did need to recognize the significance of the homonymous (non congruent) field defect reported to him and refer urgently for a neurology opinion/head scan. It was also necessary to 'safety net' by notifying the patient directly.

Dr Fowler's actions would also not be defensible on breach of duty because he should have looked at the earlier clinical note, recognized that the field defect was homonymous and referred urgently for a head scan or neurological opinion.

 Legal comment

Neither Dr Saad's, nor Dr Fowler's standard of care can be defended. If this was Jayne's claim, then a neurosurgeon would be called on to comment on whether referral 6 months previously would make any difference to her outcome. But that is not the question that is posed. The claim comes from the driver of the car who was injured in the accident.

With appropriate referral, the glioma would have been diagnosed well before the fit and treatment may have postponed the deterioration. But there is a more fundamental point. People suffering from a medical condition are under a duty to report the condition to DVLA, if it affects their ability to drive. If the condition had been diagnosed earlier, Jayne would have received advice from her doctors and she would have surrendered her driving licence. In her condition, she should not have been driving and the blame for the accident must, therefore, lie at the door of Dr Saad and Dr Fowler. Their MDOs will have to compensate the injured driver.

 Key learning points

Specific to the case

• It is important to distinguish between visual symptoms or signs that are binocular (and therefore arising posterior to the optic chiasm) and those that are uniocular (and therefore in retinal or optic nerve).

General points

• It is always necessary to take notice and gibe weight to the opinions of colleagues such as opticians, physiotherapists, osteopaths etc. They often have a great deal of experience of what is 'normal' and what is not.

• When medical errors occur there is usually a concatenation of errors by individuals. It is relatively unusual to have only a single defendant.

• Many errors occur because of communication failures. It is good practice to always 'safety net' communications with other disciplines by saying to the patient 'I am referring you to . . . if you do not hear within x weeks ring me.' It is helpful to record this advice.

Further reading and references

Hamilton W, Kernick D (2007) Clinical features of primary brain tumours: a case-control study using electronic primary care records. *BJGP* **57**: 695–9.

Steiner TJ, MacGregor EA, Davies PT (2009) Guidelines for All Healthcare Professionals in the Diagnosis and Management of Migraine, Tension-Type, Cluster and Medication-Overuse Headaches. British Association for the Study of Headaches.

Case 38 A man with a headache: Swine flu or meningitis?

A woman telephoned Dr Craig in late July 2009 on a weekend evening. She was concerned about her husband Joe, aged 42. She stated that he had been feeling unwell for three days with a fever. He had a persistent headache. He had vomited once in the bed. She said she preferred to keep the curtains shut and was feeling generally unwell.

Dr Craig, who was triaging calls, referred to an e-mail from the Royal College of GPs (July 2009) that stated:

The Department of Health advises that people who have any of the following symptoms and a temperature of 38 °C and above or feels hot may have swine flu.

The typical symptoms are:
- sudden fever (a high body temperature of 38 °C/ 100.4 °F or above), and
- sudden cough.

Other symptoms may include:
- headache,
- tiredness,
- chills,
- aching muscles,
- limb or joint pain,
- diarrhoea or stomach upset,
- sore throat,
- runny nose,
- sneezing, and
- loss of appetite

What would you do now?

Dr Craig established that there was a history of fever (over 38 °C), a headache, and muscular aching. He was told about the single vomit (about 12 hours previously). He established there was no breathing difficulty, no sore throat, no cough, or runny nose. Dr Craig suggested to Joe's wife that the diagnosis was probably swine flu. Dr Craig issued a prescription for Tamiflu.

Was it reasonable to diagnosis swine flu and authorize Tamiflu?

Five hours later Joe's wife telephoned back. Dr Craig asked her whether there was anything else that particularly concerned her or anything that seemed to her to be unusual for influenza. She responded that Joe had been unhappy with the light when she had opened the curtains, and also seemed at one point to have been uncertain as to what day it was and how long he had been ill.

What would be your differential diagnosis and how would you discriminate between them?

The information suggesting photophobia and possible confusion was a matter for concern to Dr Craig and he arranged for a colleague, Dr Evans, to visit. Dr Evans found that Joe had a fever of 38.5 °C, appeared to have a severe headache, and appeared to have pain and stiffness when Dr Evans flexed his neck. There was no evidence of mental confusion and Joe denied having been disorientated. However, Dr Evans was concerned about meningitis and referred Joe to hospital as an emergency.

In hospital Joe had a lumbar puncture which did not confirm bacterial meningitis – he was treated with antibiotics but the final conclusion was that he had a viral meningitis.

In this case Joe and his wife were grateful to Dr Evans for his prompt and accurate response.

Can Dr Craig be criticized for his initial diagnosis of flu? Headache is relatively common with influenza. How does one avoid admitting everyone with flu?

Avoiding Errors in General Practice, First Edition. Kevin Barraclough, Jenny du Toit, Jeremy Budd, Joseph E. Raine, Kate Williams and Jonathan Bonser.
© 2013 John Wiley & Sons, Ltd. Published 2013 by John Wiley & Sons, Ltd.

Expert comment

It is difficult to avoid the temptation to avoid cutting corners and making the 'obvious' diagnosis, particularly in times of an epidemic.

The familiar cognitive errors would be 'anchoring' (a reluctance to depart from the basic hypothesis that this would be a case of influenza), 'availability' (because the diagnosis of influenza would be in mind during an epidemic) and confirmation bias (a tendency to elicit symptoms consistent with the influenza hypothesis) leading to premature diagnostic closure.

In this case the coincidence of fever, headache and general malaise did suggest the diagnosis of influenza. However, there was a lack of respiratory tract symptoms. This is unusual with influenza. 84% of patients with influenza have a cough and only 16% do not (Call *et al.*, 2004). 84% of patients with influenza also have headache but photophobia and neck stiffness is rare (Call *et al.*, 2004). At the time of the second telephone consultation Dr Craig sought information that was *inconsistent* with the hypothesis of influenza and was rewarded with the mention of photophobia and possible confusion.

 Legal comment

Dr Craig's initial diagnosis of flu was wrong. Perhaps he could be criticized, because he did not arrange for Joe to be seen sooner. However, there has been no adverse outcome and Joe and his wife are grateful for the care that Dr Evans provided.

 Key learning points

General points
- It is always necessary to be wary of details that 'do not fit'.

References and further reading

Attia J, Hatala R, Cook DJ, *et al.* (1999) Does this adult patient have acute meningitis? *JAMA* **282**(2): 175–81 (doi:10.1001/jama.282.2.175)

Call SA, Vollenweider MA, Hornung CA, Simel DL, McKinney WP (2005) Does this patient have influenza? *JAMA* **293**: 987–97.

Meningitis Research Foundation. http://www.meningitis.org/

Case 39 A woman suffering dizziness

Cynthia was a 52-year-old woman who had suffered from anxiety and depression for many years. She had been under the local psychiatric services for 16 years. She requested a home visit because she was dizzy and Dr Kirby, a GP registrar, visited her at home. Dr Kirby noted that Cynthia had been unsteady on her feet for several days. She had vomited once. Examination was unremarkable other than that Cynthia's blood pressure, which dropped from a systolic of 118 mm/hg when sitting to 108 mm/hg on standing. Dr Kirby noted that Cynthia had been started on lisinopril 3 weeks earlier. She advised Cynthia to stop the lisinopril and call again if her dizziness did not improve.

Was there anything else you would have checked?

A week later Cynthia was no better and she called for another visit. Dr Clarke, Dr Kirby's trainer visited. Dr Clarke noted that Cynthia's dizziness was not postural. She felt unsteady even sitting in a chair. She had no frank vertigo but had difficulty walking in a straight line, had difficulty drinking a cup of water and appeared a little dehydrated. Dr Kirby noted that Cynthia had been taking lithium for 12 years and arranged for the district nurses to visit and take a serum lithium level.

What would be your differential diagnosis and what would you have done?

The blood lithium level was not available until the following Monday (3 days later) and came back as 1.56 mmol/l. Dr Clarke spoke to the district nurses and established that they were unsure when Cynthia had taken her lithium and therefore whether the test was more than 12 hours after the previous dose. Dr Clarke arranged for the test to be repeated with the blood test to be taken in the morning before Cynthia had taken her daily dose.

The blood test was not taken until the following Thursday. On the Thursday evening Cynthia was seen by Dr Creed from the Out of Hours service. Dr Creed noted that Cynthia was extremely agitated and anxious. She was orientated in time and place but appeared a little dehydrated, with a dry mouth and a resting pulse rate of 100 bpm. Dr Creed wondered about an anxiety disorder or thyrotoxicosis and requested that her own general practitioner visit the following day.

On the Friday morning Dr Clarke received the result that Cynthia's serum lithium level was 2.15 mmol/l. He arranged her immediate admission. She was treated for lithium toxicity and dehydration but was left with significant ataxia and dysarthria. Cynthia brought a claim against Dr Kirby and Dr Clarke alleging that Dr Kirby had missed the significance of the fact that Cynthia was taking lithium and liable to be suffering from lithium toxicity, and Dr Clarke had suspected the diagnosis but not acted with sufficient alacrity.

Do you think her claim will succeed?

 ### Expert comment

Allegations of failure to monitor drugs, failure to recognize drug toxicity and failure, in particular to monitor serum lithium levels are relatively common causes of claims against general practitioners. Other drugs that occur fairly regularly in claims about monitoring are phenytoin, azathioprine, methotrexate and amiodarone.

In most of the cases the drug will have been started by specialist services and the monitoring then delegated to general practitioners. Patients are on the drugs for many years and the drugs sometimes get overlooked. In the case of lithium toxicity the patients will always have mental health problems and may have defaulted on follow up, and then get lost. Most practices nowadays will regularly audit the few patients they have on lithium

---

Avoiding Errors in General Practice, First Edition. Kevin Barraclough, Jenny du Toit, Jeremy Budd, Joseph E. Raine, Kate Williams and Jonathan Bonser.
© 2013 John Wiley & Sons, Ltd. Published 2013 by John Wiley & Sons, Ltd.

and patients who have defaulted will be identified in that way.

Symptoms that are due to drug side effects may be particularly difficult to identify. However, the general practitioner needs to be fully aware of the high risk drugs and high risk symptoms such as breathlessness in the patient on amiodarone, nausea in the patient on azathioprine or ataxia in any drug with cerebellar side effects.

'Dizziness' is a common and difficult symptom in primary care. 'There can be few physicians so dedicated to their art that they do not experience a slight decline in spirits when they learn that their patient's complaint is giddiness' (Matthews, 1963). However, a clear history will generally distinguish postural pre syncope (only occurs on standing), frank vertigo – either sustained (possible acute vestibular neuritis) or not sustained and positional (BPPV), light-headedness when not distracted (hyperventilation) or unsteadiness on walking in the elderly, especially on the turn (disequilibrium of the elderly).

In this case one of the key features that Dr Kirby failed to identify was that Cynthia did not have vertigo or postural pre syncope but had both truncal and limb ataxia. If Cynthia had been drinking her clinical features would have been those of alcohol intoxication causing a cerebellar ataxia with cerebellar signs (rolling gait, poor heel-to-toe walking, positive Romberg's sign, and dysdodokinesis). Cynthia would probably also have been slightly dysarthric. Dr Kirby needed to recognize that, in an unsteady patient on lithium, the condition that you cannot afford to miss is lithium toxicity. The initiation of the ACE inhibitor may have been a precipitant, but once the patient is dehydrated the situation is critical.

Dr Clarke correctly identified the possibility of lithium toxicity but, possibly not unreasonably since he had never encountered it before, failed to realize that the condition is an emergency. He should really have consulted the BNF:

Overdosage, usually with serum-lithium concentration of over 1.5 mmol/litre, may be fatal and toxic effects include tremor, ataxia, dysarthria, nystagmus, renal impairment, and convulsions. If these potentially hazardous signs occur, treatment should be stopped, serum-lithium concentrations redetermined, and steps taken to reverse lithium toxicity. In mild cases withdrawal of lithium and administration of sodium salts and fluid will reverse the toxicity. A serum-lithium concentration in excess of 2 mmol/litre requires urgent treatment.

Neither of the doctors' actions would be defensible on breach of duty and the irreversible consequences of lithium toxicity are often, as in this case, very serious.

 Legal comment

Causation flows from the breach of duty. Thus the MDOs of both Dr Kirby and Dr Clarke will have to settle this claim. The value of the claim will depend on the extent of the dysarthria and ataxia, but it is likely to be several hundred thousand pounds.

The fact that Dr Kirby is a registrar does not excuse his failure. He is expected to act with the same level of competence as a fully qualified general practitioner. The registrar has immediate access to the opinion of the supervising partner and is expected to use this facility whenever it is necessary. If he was in any doubt, he should have referred the matter to his trainer, Dr Clarke. This would have perhaps exonerated him to some extent, but it would not have altered the outcome. We already know that Dr Clarke did not cover himself with glory, when he saw Cynthia.

 Key learning points

Specific to the case
- It is extremely important to be aware of the clinical features of lithium toxicity in a patient taking lithium.
- Lithium toxicity is a medical emergency as the consequences, particularly if exacerbated by dehydration, can be death or irreversible neurological or renal damage.
- It is important not to mistake ataxia for other causes of 'dizziness'. It helps to remember that the features are generally those of alcohol intoxication.

General points
- Always look at the drugs the patient is taking and consider if they are causing or contributing to the symptoms.

References and further reading

Barraclough K, Adolfo Bronstein (2009) Diagnosis in general practice: vertigo. *BMJ*, **339**: 749–52.

Matthews WB (1963) *Practical Neurology*. Oxford: Blackwell.

Case 40 A middle-aged man with an ankle injury

Paul was 45 years old when he saw Dr du Vivier about an injury to his right foot/ankle area which he had sustained playing badminton three days earlier. He had felt something go bang in his calf and thought his opponent had hit him. Dr du Vivier examined Paul, noted the history, recorded there was some slight calf swelling and 'achilles tendon intact' and diagnosed a calf muscle strain.

What other information would you obtain in a case such as this?

Three weeks later Paul consulted Dr Prasad. Dr Prasad agreed with Dr du Vivier's assessment and prescribed exercises and naproxen. Two weeks later Paul was still having difficulty walking. He attended A&E. An orthopaedic registrar diagnosed a complete Achilles tendon rupture.

Paul underwent an attempted tendon repair a week later but brought an action against Dr du Vivier and Dr Prasad for failing to diagnose the injury. It was alleged that the general practitioners had not carried out a 'calf squeeze test' or asked Paul to stand on tiptoe. Dr du Vivier claimed that he had asked Paul to stand on tiptoe but agreed that he had not done a 'calf squeeze test'.

Do you think a claim against the GP will succeed?

 Expert comment

In this case there was no dispute that the patient had given the 'classic' history of an acute onset of pain leading to the (incorrect) belief he had been struck from behind. With this history the diagnosis of Achilles tendon rupture has to be excluded and accordingly Dr du Vivier's failure to carry out a more specific test could not be defended.

Specific tests should include Simmond's test (sometimes known as a Thompson test). The test is probably better described as the 'calf squeeze' test. With the patient kneeling, squeezing the calf should cause passive plantar flexion. If the tendon is ruptured plantar flexion is diminished or absent (the degree of movement of the foot can be compared with the other side). Significant asymmetry of movement is also very suggestive of rupture.

Another commonly used test is to ask the patient to stand on tip toes. Dr du Vivier claimed that he had carried out this test. Because the Achilles tendon transmits the main force of plantar flexion, a patient with a rupture will be unable to stand on tiptoe on that side. However, a difficulty about relying completely on the (bilateral) 'tiptoe' test is that the patient maybe taking the majority of the weight on the uninjured side.

The cause of the error in this case can probably be characterized as a simple lack of knowledge. Achilles tendon rupture is not commonly seen in UK general practice (perhaps one case every 7 or 8 years). Many GPs do not experience orthopaedic surgery or Accident and Emergency in their training and the subject is not extensively discussed in nonspecialist orthopaedic texts.

The examination of Dr du Vivier was limited to palpation of the tendon and (as a fact disputed by the claimant) asking Paul to stand on tiptoe. Palpation of the tendon is not guaranteed to detect all tendon ruptures because swelling and haematoma can disguise the gap. Equally, a patient may be able to stand on (bilateral) tiptoe by taking the weight on the uninjured side.

Missed rupture of the Achilles tendon causes quite significant disability compared to early diagnosis and consequently these cases can be quite expensive for the medical defence organizations.

Avoiding Errors in General Practice, First Edition. Kevin Barraclough, Jenny du Toit, Jeremy Budd, Joseph E. Raine, Kate Williams and Jonathan Bonser.
© 2013 John Wiley & Sons, Ltd. Published 2013 by John Wiley & Sons, Ltd.

Legal comment

This failure to diagnose cannot be defended and the claim must be settled as soon as possible. Early diagnosis is the key to a good outcome. Thus it may be that by the time Dr Prasad saw Paul three and a half weeks after the injury, it was too late to alter the outcome. If so and if Dr Prasad and Dr du Vivier belong to different MDOs, then Dr Prasad's MDO will deny responsibility and refuse to contribute to the settlement. Whether they will avoid contributing altogether depends on the orthopaedic evidence the MDOs receive.

 Key learning points

Specific to the case
• 20–25% of Achilles tendon ruptures are missed at first presentation. The classic history is of a sudden injury associated with sporting activity.

• With a possible Achilles tendon injury always check the calf squeeze test (compare foot plantar flexion with the other side) and ask the patient to stand on tip toes.
• Abnormalities of these tests occur in almost all cases of Achilles tendon rupture. The tests have a high sensitivity and a negative result rules the condition out (a SnOUT).

General points
• Good 'SnOUT' tests are not common and should be used gratefully!

Further reading

NHS Clinical knowledge summaries http://www.patient.co.uk/doctor/Achilles-Tendonitis-and-Rupture.htm

PART 3

Investigating and dealing with errors

1 Introduction

Part 1 of this book looked at how errors occur. Part 2 examined detailed examples of errors. This third section looks at the mechanisms in place to pick up and then respond to errors. Those mechanisms are operated by the organization providing the healthcare (e.g. by the Primary Care Trust or the medical practice itself), by the professional regulatory system (NCAS, the GMC), and by the wider legal system (the Coroner, the civil or criminal Courts).

A doctor who makes an error may find himself the subject of investigations by each of these bodies. For example the doctors in the vincristine case referred to in section 1 will have no doubt faced internal hospital investigations with a view to disciplinary proceedings.

There was certainly a police investigation and it led to a criminal trial. The death of the patient was reported to the Coroner and an Inquest was opened. The family of the patient may well have sued the hospital for damages for its negligence. The case will also certainly have come to the attention of the GMC.

Rightly or wrongly, the fact is that all these investigations will have primarily focused on how those individual doctors were to blame for what happened, and only secondarily on the defects in the system which may have contributed to the outcome.

This section gives a factual account of how these mechanisms work. We also give some practical advice. However, a doctor facing an investigation of any significance will need considerable legal and moral support, as we explain below.

2 How errors and their recurrence are prevented in primary care

The following are the main mechanisms for picking up errors. They are themselves subject to continuous review and discussion.

Avoiding Errors in General Practice, First Edition. Kevin Barraclough, Jenny du Toit, Jeremy Budd, Joseph E. Raine, Kate Williams and Jonathan Bonser.
© 2013 John Wiley & Sons, Ltd. Published 2013 by John Wiley & Sons, Ltd.

Guidelines and protocols

Guidelines are systematically developed statements designed to help doctors make the right healthcare decisions. They should be statements of best practice based on a review of the current medical evidence. They should summarize the key information on a topic and should be reviewed at agreed intervals to ensure that they remain up to date and have taken into account new developments. Guidelines may be national, e.g. from NICE, or they may be issued by local organizations and adapted to suit local conditions, populations and facilities. They provide a general framework for treating patients and aim to reduce variations in practice. A doctor can treat them as a useful source of reference, but ultimately he is not required to adhere strictly to them.

The term 'protocol' suggests a more rigid set of statements allowing little or no flexibility or variation. They provide the doctor with a precise sequence of activities to follow in the management of a specific condition. However, in practice, the terms 'guidelines' and 'protocols' are often used interchangeably.

Guidelines and protocols may need to be adjusted to meet individual circumstances. A doctor should always use his clinical judgment. However, any reasons for deviating from a guideline or protocol should be discussed with a senior doctor and carefully recorded in the patient's notes.

Guidelines and protocols can help a doctor make fewer mistakes. He does not need to rely solely on his memory. They can be particularly useful when a doctor faces a stressful situation. Online versions avoid problems of paper copies being lost and are easier to update. They can be particularly helpful for trainees and for doctors facing an unusual situation. A review of an adverse incident can highlight the need to create a new guideline for a particular condition in order to prevent an error recurring.

Audit

Audit is the process of comparing current practice with gold standards for best practice (these can be local, national or international). The audit cycle is a process of collecting data, comparing it with gold standards and then identifying any deficiencies in practice or areas for improvement. Changes should then be implemented and the audit repeated. It should be a continuous process to ensure that standards are continuously monitored with the overall aim of improving the quality of care. So, for example, a certain number of medical records might be reviewed on a monthly basis, so that improvements can be tracked over time.

All General Practices should have audit programmes with regular audit meetings. Protocols and guidelines often provide standards for audit.

The role of audit is to promote best practice, but in so doing it may identify areas of error. It is a key component of clinical governance and hence is a tool for minimizing harm as well as maximizing quality.

The aim is to identify priority areas for patient safety improvements.

Appraisals

All general practitioners are required to undergo an annual appraisal. For trainees, there is a separate system organized by the Deanery, which has many similarities. The appraisal should be private and confidential. Ideally, the appraiser will have been trained in the appraisal process. Appraisal is based on the GMC's booklet 'Good Medical Practice' which describes the principles of good medical practice, and the standards of competence and conduct required of doctors in their professional work. The appraisal forces doctors to think about their achievements and failings in the previous year and to consider what they would like to accomplish in the forthcoming year. As well as dealing with issues such as the doctor's clinical performance and effectiveness over the previous year, the appraisal also looks at complaints (which should be reflected on and learnt from), disciplinary matters, probity, health, continuing medical education and audit. Once completed, the appraiser and appraisee sign the form so that they are aware of any relevant issues, e.g. additional clinical training or disciplinary issues, which may require further action.

Over recent years a new type of appraisal called a 360 degree appraisal has also been introduced by some PCTs. This appraisal involves getting anonymous feedback on a doctor's performance from 10–15 colleagues (doctors, nurses, secretaries). Anonymous feedback is also obtained from 20–30 patients using set forms. Many doctors find it a very useful means of assessing their performance. It complements the standard appraisal process. In time it may become incorporated into it.

An annual appraisal will also be required as part of a doctor's GMC revalidation process (see The GMC in future (a) Revalidation below).

Complaints management

Every general practice should have a written complaints procedure which can readily be supplied to patients. Many practices publish theirs on their website.

The procedure should outline processes and timescales for both raising and responding to a complaint. For example, a complaint should usually be acknowledged within 48 hours, and a substantive response supplied within 10 days.

Complaints may be made formally and in writing, or they may be verbal and more informal. In either case, the Practice Manager should use his or her judgement on the best way to respond – and the complaints procedure should be phrased to allow for as much flexibility as possible. For example, a verbal complaint may sometimes be best dealt with by telephone or in a meeting, rather than in a letter. Many complaints are about straightforward administrative problems, such as a surgery running late or a delay obtaining an appointment, and can be dealt with very promptly. An apology is often enough. Even in such straightforward cases, though, it is important to make a record of the complaint and the resolution.

In more formal or complex cases which will take longer to investigate, patients (or their family) need to be told clearly when they can expect to receive a substantive response. Most complaints procedures allow ten days. But if that proves not to be possible, then they should be told of the delay and the reasons for it.

In more complex cases the practice manager may have to take on the role of investigator and must bring an independent mind to bear on the issues. When there are clinical issues, it can help to appoint an independent clinician to review the medical records and discuss the case with the doctor concerned and possibly the other doctors in the practice too. An honest appraisal of the merits needs to be made because, if not successfully resolved, a complaint can become litigation or even a GMC case. For those reasons, it can sometimes be helpful to get the help of an MDO adviser on the contents of a response to a complaint. It can be very important to ensure that, as well as being accurate, the tone of the response is appropriate.

The response should always conclude that the complainant can contact the Practice Manager directly if he or she is dissatisfied or does not understand. A meeting, whether just with the Practice Manager or with the doctors as well, can often go a long way to resolving misunderstandings or anxieties. It can even help to thank the patient for bringing the problem to the practice's attention.

If the complainant remains dissatisfied, he or she should be informed of their rights to take the complaint to the PCT's complaints officer or to the Health Service Ombudsman (see below).

Significant Event Analysis

Significant Event Analysis (SEA) is a structured way of investigating incidents, and is comparable to the Root Cause Analysis used in hospitals. Its use is now a requirement of the NHS contract and is a part of GP appraisals. It is intended to ensure a review of the wider picture of the causes of events, and to capture what has been learnt from the incident and what changes have been made as a result.

3   The role of the Primary Care Trusts

At the time of writing, Primary Care Trusts are being gradually disbanded in favour of GP Commissioning bodies. PCTs have had a significant role in the management and regulation of primary care services, and it is not yet clear what organization will take on those functions in the future. Current expectations are that the National Commissioning Board will take over the management of a single national Performers' List to ensure that only 'performers' of an acceptable standard are allowed to practise in primary care. What follows is a description of the current arrangements, which are likely to be adapted but probably not significantly changed in the relatively near future.

Performers' Lists

Standards of performance in NHS primary care for the last eight years have been regulated through Performers' Lists, held by local Primary Care Trusts. At present, every doctor wishing to practise in NHS primary care must apply to have his name included in a local list. Inclusion in one list in England will entitle him to practise in any PCT in England. In Wales, Scotland and Northern Ireland, local Health Boards have separate lists operated under different rules.

An application must include a lot of information about the doctor, including declarations as to any criminal record, any adverse outcomes of investigations into past professional conduct, as well as any current investigations. References from recent posts must be provided.

The NHS (Performers' List) Regulations 2004 set out detailed grounds on which an application can be refused by the PCT. The most important are that the applicant is not 'suitable' (which usually means he has a criminal record) or that his admission to the list would be 'prejudicial to the efficiency of the services offered by those on the list' (which means that his performance is considered below standard). In some cases, rather than an outright refusal, an applicant is accepted onto a list subject to conditions. Typically, the conditions would require a measure of supervision of the doctor's work.

Once on the list, a 'performer' can be removed by the PCT on various grounds, but in particular his 'unsuitability' or his 'inefficiency'. Another ground for removal is that the performer has not actually worked in the area of the PCT for the last twelve months. (For this reason, it is important that doctors who work in several locations should keep in touch with their 'home' PCT.)

Because the effect of removal can devastate a doctor's livelihood, the Performers' List rules provide basic safeguards for fairness and 'natural justice'. So, the PCT must always give the doctor due notice of the allegation against him which is under consideration, and of the measures now being sought by the PCT. As an alternative to outright removal, the PCT might want what is called a 'contingent removal' (meaning that conditions are placed on his inclusion on the list). Or it may want the doctor to be nationally disqualified (meaning that he cannot apply for inclusion on any PCT list).

Faced with a notice from his PCT, the doctor has the right to either make representations in writing or (and probably more appropriately) he can call for an oral hearing to look into the allegation. That hearing will take place before a panel of three people appointed by the PCT.

In these circumstances, the doctor should certainly consult his MDO for advice and support in the conduct of the case. If the case is of some complexity, or if it involves cross-examination of witnesses, the doctor may well have grounds to insist on a legally qualified advocate to present his case. Furthermore, before the hearing it is sometimes possible to negotiate for agreed conditions rather than removal, so that the PCT will then cancel the hearing altogether. The MDOs will advise on this, and sometimes will conduct negotiations on behalf of the doctor.

A PCT can also seek a doctor's suspension from the list as a temporary measure to protect the public while other investigations are being conducted. For example, a doctor awaiting a trial in a criminal case, or who has a GMC hearing pending can find himself suspended from the list and unable to work in primary care until the main case is concluded. Depending on the outcome of the main case, there could then be proceedings for his removal from the list.

There is an appeal process for all these various Performers' List decisions. Appeals go to what is known as the First Tier Tribunal, which has its own judicial processes which are overseen by a judge.

4   Other investigations

National Clinical Assessment Service (NCAS)

NCAS was established in 2001. Its purpose is to advise healthcare organizations (both NHS and private) which have concerns about the practice of doctors, dentists or pharmacists for whom they are responsible. Its aim is to help those organizations look quickly and fairly into questions about the performance or conduct of a doctor or other healthcare professional.

A referring organization (in the case of general practitioners, usually a PCT) can contact a NCAS adviser who will then talk through a case and advise on how to investigate further, whether to consider excluding a doctor and/or whether to implement Performers' List action. Advice given on the telephone will usually then be confirmed in writing. (Copies of correspondence will, in principle, be disclosable to the doctor under the Data Protection Act.) As the case develops, the NCAS adviser will continue to advise as required. NCAS reports that over the ten years of its existence, requests for help have increased tenfold from about 100 in its first year, to more than 1000 in 2010.

In addition to advising, NCAS will, upon request, provide clinical assessment services. An assessment of a doctor's competence cannot be carried out without his agreement. (The idea will be presented to him as the alternative to something worse, e.g. Performers' List action or a GMC referral.) An assessment might be directed towards clinical concerns, health concerns, 'communicative competence' and/or behaviour concerns. NCAS reports that about one referral in twenty will involve a clinical assessment. Its published statistics show that the medical specialty most likely to be assessed is general medical practice, and that older practitioners are more likely to be assessed than younger ones.

The clinical assessment process is wide ranging and includes an occupational health assessment, a behavioural assessment, and a clinical assessment visit. There will be assessment workbook exercises and feedback from patients and peers.

The assessment will conclude with a report setting out the findings based on triangulated evidence (i.e. evidence from three different sources) and recommending the next step for both the doctor and the referrer. This will usually be a structured action plan, involving the monitoring of the doctor's performance with clear points identified at which the situation is to be reviewed.

Last year (2010/2011) the assessment process ended with three out of every four practitioners assessed continuing to do clinical work, albeit nearly half of them with some kind of restriction on their practice.

The most common clinical issues that NCAS deals with are child protection issues, prescribing and diagnostic skills. The most common behavioural problem is communication with colleagues.

In some cases of serious concern, NCAS and the referring Trust may have discussions with the GMC. Indeed, advice may be given by NCAS to the PCT on referring a case to the GMC.

From the doctor's point of view, the drawback to NCAS is that its advice is based only on what it is told by the referring organization. NCAS does not conduct its own investigation into matters save when a clinical assessment is requested. Furthermore, once its advice has been given, the referring organization is highly likely to feel professionally obliged to follow it. Yet, because it is only advice, a doctor has no legal recourse against NCAS.

It is planned that NCAS will become 'self-funded' over the next few years. It seems that its customers (healthcare organizations) may have to pay for advice in the future. An aggrieved practitioner might feel, on the basis of the principle that he who pays the piper calls the tune, that NCAS may then become even less impartial.

Partnership issues arising from errors

In civil law, partners are jointly and severally liable for each others' actions. For example, a GP who assaults a patient in the course of his work is personally responsible for his actions in criminal law and to the GMC. But if the assaulted patient seeks compensation, then not only is that doctor responsible, but so are each and every one of his partners.

The need for the partners to have indemnity against such claims is obvious in principle, but can easily be overlooked in practice. Partnership agreements often provide that it is for each individual partner to arrange their own cover with an MDO. But to guard against the possibility that one of them defaults without the others knowing, it is advisable for partnerships to centrally supervise and manage the cover arrangements for each doctor, and deduct the subscriptions from their partnership drawings.

Where a partner's performance appears to be slipping, the other partners may be concerned about their own personal liability for his errors and also about the risk posed to the reputation of the practice. What can they do about it?

The answer is that it depends on whether the partnership is governed by a binding partnership agreement and, if so, what its terms are. A well-drawn partnership agreement will provide the other partners with the opportunity to expel or suspend a wrong doing or poorly performing partner.

Some agreements provide for the possibility of expelling one partner on the unanimous votes of the others, even where that partner has done nothing wrong at all. Known as a 'green sock' clause (i.e. one which allows expulsion for nothing more than the notional sin of wearing green socks), this clause can mean the removal of a partner without any investigation into whether or not he has actually done wrong. To this extent, his rights are less than those of an employee.

Other partnership agreements will provide a list of circumstances where expulsion is justified. Examples would be breaching the terms of the partnership agreement, breaching medical ethics, committing a crime or being struck off the medical register. The expulsion must be carried out in accordance with a specified procedure. This will probably mean a special notice of a meeting for that purpose, and a specified majority voting in favour. The partnership agreement will probably provide for an appeal process by which to challenge the expulsion. Usually this will be by the appointment of an independent arbitrator, who will want to see some evidence that the circumstances did indeed justify taking this action under the partnership agreement. Depending on the terms of the Partnership Agreement, the expelled partner may or may not continue as a partner until the arbitration is concluded and be entitled to receive drawings until that time.

In a surprisingly large number of cases, a medical practice has no binding agreement governing its relations with each other in the partnership. In that case, they will have been operating as a 'partnership at will' and the partners have fewer options. They can either persuade the wrongdoing partner to leave or they can dissolve the partnership completely. As dissolution would usually constitute a disaster for the business of the partnership (since it jeopardizes its contract with the PCT to provide medical services), the wrongdoing partner will be in a relatively strong negotiating position.

GPs in partnership would be well advised to check regularly on the validity of their Partnership Agreement.

The Care Quality Commission

The Care Quality Commission regulates health and social care services in the public and private sectors to ensure that they meet essential standards. It covers a wide range of organizations, including hospitals, care homes and dentists. All these organizations must register, and are then subject to inspections (announced or unannounced) and reports. The Commission has powers of enforcement and can impose fines and warnings and even suspend the operation of an organization.

From 2012, GP practices will be included in the CQC's remit, and must register. It is intended that they are inspected approximately every two years on an announced basis.

The 'essential standards' are concerned with ensuring a safe and clean environment, that patients are treated with respect and dignity and that staff are appropriately managed.

5 Legal advice – where to get it and how to pay

If, despite a doctor's best intentions and endeavours, he finds himself on the wrong end of a complaint or an investigation, such as we have described in this section, he is likely to be catapulted from the more or less comfortable and familiar environment of community medical practice into an alien, possibly hostile world, very different from his usual work experience. This is a world governed by legal rules, deadlines and procedures. The doctor will need assistance to guide him through this unfamiliar territory. Colleagues may offer advice and, for more minor complaints, this may be enough. But if the complaint is at all serious, then he will require access to legal advice. After all, a complaint could be the beginning of a process which will end with limits on the doctor's ability to practise, the payment of damages, (which could even run to millions of pounds), and a requirement to pay the legal costs incurred by the patient or the family. Then there are the legal costs incurred by the lawyers representing the individual doctor or the clinical team. The level of these costs will usually be based on the time spent on the case, but bills of tens of thousands of pounds would not be unusual for a case of moderate complexity.

Who pays these legal bills? The answer depends on factors including the nature of the initial complaint, whether or not the general practitioner has membership of an MDO or other insurance cover.

(a) Negligence claims

All doctors employed in NHS hospitals or directly employed by PCTs are covered for claims against them through the NHS's indemnity scheme. This means that the payment of both damages and bills for legal advice in respect of claims will be organized through the National Health Service Litigation Authority (NHSLA) in England, Welsh Health Legal Services in Wales, the individual Health Boards and Trusts in Northern Ireland and the Central Legal Office in Scotland. These bodies will organize legal representation and make decisions about the conduct of the case. The general practitioner involved in the treatment of the patient will be expected to cooperate with the lawyers appointed by these public health bodies to defend the interests of the NHS trust.

However, most general practitioners are either employed by or a partner in a medical practice. They may work as self employed locums. They are not covered under the NHS indemnity scheme. Instead they should be covered by Medical Defence Organizations (MDOs) – mostly the Medical Protection Society, Medical Defence Union or the Medical and Dental Defence Union of Scotland. Unlike hospital doctors, the vast majority of general medical practitioners, whether working in the private sector or the NHS, need their own cover against a claim for medical negligence.

(b)   Other enquiries

A general practitioner facing any of the investigations in to his clinical practice as described in this section may well be able to get legal advice and support from his MDO. Support may be declined if the MDO considers that the matters in question arise not so much from clinical practice as from personal conduct. Furthermore, MDOs do not usually provide support to members for partnership disputes, regarding them as more in the nature of commercial or business matters which are outside their protection.

Medical Defence Organizations

General practitioners have even more need than hospital based doctors for cover against the consequences of their errors.

Until recently there were only three indemnity organizations offering legal assistance to doctors in the United Kingdom, namely the Medical Protection Society (MPS), the Medical Defence Union (MDU), and the Medical and Dental Defence Union of Scotland (MDDUS). Now there are a number of other options, but these three organizations still look after the interests of the vast majority of UK general practitioners. There are variations in the kinds of indemnity they offer, from insurance based cover to discretionary cover or a combination of the two. The doctor looking for MDO cover must look carefully at the terms and discuss them with the MDO in order to decide what kind of cover best suits him. The MDO websites each give a brief account of what is on offer.

Whatever their differences, in essence, the MDOs offer members professional and legal advice. If a doctor is a member of one of these organizations, then subject to the terms of his cover, he can call on that organization to come to his assistance in his time of need. All the MDOs offer telephone helplines, whereby a clinician can talk to a medico-legal advisor on professional matters of concern, small or large. They lend a kindly ear.

To establish which cover is most appropriate, we strongly recommend that doctors contact the MDOs to find out their terms and what they mean in theory and in practice.

6 External inquiries

The Health Service Ombudsman

A complainant may not be satisfied with the outcome of a complaint. In that case the GP practice will tell him of his right to ask the Health Service Commissioner ('HSC', often known as the 'Health Service Ombudsman'), to investigate. This is the last port of call for a person with a complaint about NHS services.

A complainant can only approach the Ombudsman when the local complaints procedure has been concluded. The function of the Ombudsman is, upon request, and at his/her discretion to investigate an alleged injustice or hardship caused by a failure in administration or service in the NHS.

If the Ombudsman takes on the case (and he/she does not have to do so) he/she has powers to call for relevant documents to be produced. Arrangements will be made for the main protagonists to be interviewed. The interviewees will be sent copies of their interview notes. The general practitioner will be sent a copy of the draft report, and given the opportunity to comment on it. In practice, the report will go through several drafts before it is concluded.

The report will comment on the standard of care and service found in the particular case. The Ombudsman cannot *require* any specific steps to be taken to remedy any hardship. He/she can only make recommendations. However those recommendations do have a strong moral force, particularly given the power to 'name and shame'. Furthermore, a failure by a doctor to comply may lead to his referral to the GMC. Generally, apologies or explanations to the complainant and/or payment of money as compensation will be recommended. The Ombudsman may recommend ways to improve the service found to be at fault. The current Ombudsman (Anne Abrahams) has recently published a high-profile report called 'Care and Compassion' reciting her findings at a number of NHS institutions following complaints about poor care for the elderly. It can be seen that, as resources in the NHS are pruned down, the Ombudsman could play an important role in setting and maintaining standards of provision.

When the role of Health Service Ombudsman was first established, consideration of questions of clinical judgement by an individual doctor were specifically excluded from his remit. This has subsequently changed, and so the Ombudsman can and does now comment on the clinical judgements made by individual doctors, especially when an issue is whether those judgements have led to injustice and hardship. The Ombudsman will usually appoint Independent Assessors from the relevant medical speciality to advise on such questions. The conclusion on such questions will be based both on the facts and on the relevant professional standards (i.e. for doctors the *Bolam test* as described in Section 1).

Once concluded, the report is put before Parliament. It is also available on the Internet. It is in the public domain. A doctor who is exposed to the risk of criticism in this report may be well advised to ask his MDO for support in corresponding with the Ombudsman before it is published. Once published, his only recourse is by way of Judicial Review in the High Court, which may possibly provide a remedy if the Ombudsman's reasoning is significantly faulty or he has exceeded his remit.

Negligence claims and the litigation process

If a patient or the patient's family issues a claim against a GP about his treatment, then the doctor's MDO will instruct solicitors to investigate the claim and to defend it, if that is appropriate. The solicitors will deal with the day-to-day management of the case, responding to correspondence from the family's legal team and attending procedural hearings at Court. They will keep the MDO and the doctor himself abreast of developments. One of the roles of the solicitor acting on behalf of a clinician is to minimize the worry for him.

In practical terms, a doctor's initial involvement in a claim will be a meeting with the solicitor to discuss his treatment of the patient. The solicitor will normally draft a statement summarizing that treatment and will ask the doctor to approve its contents. This will be used to obtain expert opinion on the case. The solicitor may send the doctor various documents, such as the medical records, witness statements, the reports of the experts for the doctor and those for the claimant. He may ask for comments on these documents.

If the case appears defensible, then the legal team will wish to test the evidence and will arrange a conference with Counsel, i.e. a meeting with a barrister. The doctor will normally be required to attend such a meeting. The barrister will question him closely on his treatment of the patient and ask the experts to comment on that treatment. It may be that the legal team will need two or three conferences before a final decision is made to defend the case in Court or to reach a settlement with the claimant. In rough terms, it will probably take three years from the first notification of the claim until a case comes to trial. However, the vast majority of claims are settled before trial, in some cases because the claimant withdraws or in others because the defendant makes an offer.

Negligence claims make only a relative small call on a doctor's time. In the case of a general practitioner, the damages and costs payable to the family should come or from the coffers of an MDO. Such claims do not attract any sanction in themselves to affect a doctor's ability to work as a doctor.

Coroner's Court

In England, Wales and Northern Ireland, where there is a sudden death of which the cause is unknown, where there has been a violent or unnatural death, or where there has been a death in custody, the case has to be referred to the Coroner for an inquest, or inquiry. (In Scotland, there is a different procedure, which we describe below.)

The Coroner's role is to answer four simple factual questions:

1. Who died?
2. When did he or she die?
3. Where did he or she die?
4. How did he or she die?

In practice, it is the latter question which tends to occupy the Coroner's time. When he explores this question, it is important to understand that, in principle, he is not allowed to ask questions which tend to ascribe blame or responsibility. He should restrict himself to the bare facts. In practice, however, the question of how someone died often tends to raise just such questions.

The Coroner will gather evidence from most of those involved. His enquiries will be assisted by the expert opinion of the pathologist who carries out the post-mortem examination. He may also seek other expert opinion, medical or nonmedical, to help him reach a conclusion.

If you are asked to assist a Coroner's enquiry, you will be asked to provide a report outlining your involvement. As this will be read not only by the Coroner, but also possibly by the other witnesses, it may be important to seek advice about it. If you have any concerns about an inquest you should seek advice from your MDO which will help you prepare.

Unless the Coroner decides, having looked at the papers, that the death was, after all, a natural one which he has no duty to investigate, he will hold a public hearing by way of investigation. Witnesses, including the doctors involved, may be called to give evidence.

The Coroner's Court is not like other courts. It is not an adversarial procedure, no one is on trial, there are no sides or parties, and no prosecution or defence. Instead, there are just persons with an interest in the proceedings. These characteristics are unique in the English legal system and of ancient origin.

The Coroner runs the Court. Thus all witnesses are called by the Coroner and he asks them most of the questions. The Coroner directs the case, which is driven by his opinion. In certain limited circumstances, such as a death in custody, a jury is required to hear the evidence and reach a verdict.

Others with an interest in the proceedings, such as the family or the hospital, also get an opportunity to ask questions of witnesses. The Coroner must ensure that only questions which are relevant to the inquest are put to the witnesses, that is to say, relevant to the four factual matters he is required to investigate.

It is, however, sometimes the case that the family of the deceased feels someone, or some organization (such as a hospital) is to blame for the death. They see the inquest as an opportunity to explore and expose that fault. While, in principle, the Coroner is not allowed to make findings of fault, the question 'how' someone died often does beg the question of fault. For example, if someone dies unexpectedly, the investigation may focus on how a delay in treatment contributed to the death. In addition, the Coroner has the power to make a finding of 'neglect' in certain extreme cases of a total failure to provide basic care and attention when it was obviously required. The family may ask the Coroner to make such a finding, for example, in a case where a doctor failed to visit when a visit was clearly required.

For a doctor, it is an obvious occupational hazard that a patient might die unexpectedly. If a doctor is only asked to attend an inquest once or twice in his career, he will have been fortunate. He is likely to feel uncomfortable anyway, but especially if he knows the case is a contentious one. In those cases, it may be appropriate for an individual doctor to have his own lawyer at the inquest to look after his interests. The MDO will give advice on this situation, and if appropriate, will instruct a lawyer.

Having heard the evidence, the Coroner (or perhaps the jury) will deliver his 'verdict'. Traditionally, this was limited to death by natural causes, or accident or misadventure (which means an unintended consequence of an intentional act – an example would be a surgical mishap), suicide, unlawful killing or an open verdict (to name the most common). As already mentioned, the Coroner might add a rider of 'neglect' to some verdicts. This is a finding any general practitioner will be at pains to avoid.

Instead of the traditional brief verdict, there is now a trend for coroners to return a 'narrative verdict'. This is a short factual summary, usually only four or five lines long. It is meant to give an outcome for the family which is more satisfactory than the standard words.

Inquests are held in public, and there are often reports of them in the local or even national press. Furthermore, as a result of the evidence he has heard, the Coroner may announce at the conclusion of the inquest that he intends to make a report to a relevant authority with the power to take action to prevent the recurrence of a similar fatality to that just investigated. In an extreme case, he may report a doctor to the GMC and or to the police. Accordingly, it is important that the doctor prepares his evidence carefully.

Fatal Accident Inquiries

In Scotland, there is a different procedure for investigating the circumstances of a death. Under the Fatal Accident and Sudden Death Inquiry (Scotland) Act 1976, the Procurator Fiscal can decide to investigate any death which is sudden, suspicious, unexplained or which occurred in circumstances that give rise to serious public concern. Some investigations are mandatory, namely cases of death following an accident at work. In a minority of these investigations, the Procurator Fiscal will call for a hearing, called a Fatal Accident Inquiry. That hearing takes place before a Sheriff in the Sheriff Court. Acting in the public interest, the Procurator Fiscal will present the evidence. Other interested parties may be represented by lawyers (and often are). The Sheriff must determine:

1. where and when the death took place;
2. the cause of death;
3. any reasonable precautions whereby the death might have been avoided;
4. any defects in the system of working which contributed to the death;
5. any other relevant circumstances.

Unlike the Coroner's proceedings, questions of fault are very much in issue in these proceedings, which are therefore often quite high-profile.

Criminal matters

Sometimes things can go very badly wrong. A patient may make an allegation against a doctor of a crime, perhaps of fraud or perhaps of indecency. A patient may die unexpectedly shortly after receiving treatment. In these cases, the matter may be passed to the police to investigate.

Initially the police will take an overview. They will have to obtain evidence to support the allegation. This might be a post-mortem report, or if it is an allegation from a patient, then a statement from the patient concerned.

Then the police will want to speak to the doctor.

It cannot be stressed sufficiently how important it is for the doctor to seek advice and assistance if he knows or suspects that there is or may be a police investigation.

The police do not have 'chats', even though that is what they might call it when they contact the doctor. In fact the doctor will be interviewed under caution and that discussion will be recorded.

The police station interview will, by its very nature, be an alien, unfamiliar and intimidating experience. The police now have the power to arrest whenever they feel it is necessary. The doctor's definition of 'necessary' is likely to be different from theirs. In short, if a doctor is to be interviewed, he should anticipate that he may well be arrested.

Proper preparation for any interview with the police is vital. It is often said that cases are not won at the police station stage, but they can certainly be lost if the foundation of the doctor's case is insufficiently robust.

Preparation may include requesting a second post-mortem. It will certainly include lengthy meetings between the doctor and his legal and medical defence team, to analyze in depth the doctor's recollection of events. In most cases, a statement will be prepared to help the doctor and act as an aide-memoire in the interview. In many cases, the doctor will be advised to simply read the statement and answer no further questions.

At the start of the interview, the doctor will be 'cautioned'. This is the form of words used to ensure the police can record anything he says in answer to their questions. The words of the caution are, 'You do not have to say anything, but it may harm your defence if you do not mention when questioned something which you later rely on in court. Anything you do say may be given in evidence.' The effect of this is that the doctor's initial account must be as comprehensive as possible. The Court could make adverse inferences about any future additions to his account, for example when he gives evidence at trial.

Thankfully, most police officers realize that doctors are busy professionals. They will try to arrange a mutually convenient time for him to attend the police station. However some officers still like the dawn raid. Even if this happens, the doctor is entitled to representation. He should try to contact his MDO, but if that fails there is always a duty solicitor available to assist.

Following the interview, there will be a period of waiting. The police will have other enquiries and when they are complete they will have to seek advice from their own lawyers at the Crown Prosecution Service (CPS). The more complex the case, the longer the waiting. In the more complex manslaughter cases the waiting can even run to a couple of years.

The prosecution has to prove, so that the jury is sure of guilt, both that the act happened and the mental element of the offence. The mental element is usually (but not always) that you intended to do what is alleged. However, the charge of Gross Negligence Manslaughter is slightly different. For this charge, the jury has four questions to decide

1. Was there a duty of care?
2. Was that duty breached?
3. Did the breach cause the death? And
4. Was the negligence so 'gross' that it was criminal?

If everything goes well, the doctor will in due course be told that there is no further action. That is the end of the police investigation. However, the PCT could still investigate and the police are very likely to pass their file to the GMC, which will conduct its own investigation.

If it does not go well, the doctor will be charged. Whilst all criminal cases start in the Magistrates Court, those involving doctors are often more serious and so will be transferred to the Crown Court for trial. Any trial could be many months in the future. In the meantime, the PCT and the GMC may each take action in the interim to restrict or suspend the doctor's ability to practise.

In any dealings with the police or Courts, remember paragraph 58 of Good Medical Practice (GMP). This states:

> you must inform the GMC **without delay** [emphasis added] if, anywhere in the world you have accepted a caution, **been charged with** [emphasis added] or found guilty of a criminal offence . . .

However, and somewhat confusingly, the caution given at the beginning of an interview is different from the 'caution' one might receive as a penalty for a minor offence. At paragraph 58 of GMP, the GMC requires the penalty of a caution to be reported, *not* the one given during a police interview.

As an alternative to either a caution or a charge, the police may issue a fixed penalty notice. Such notices can now be issued for a wide range of matters, not just speeding and parking offences. Once again, somewhat confusingly, whether or not you have to report these to the GMC depends upon whether they are 'upper' or 'lower' tier matters. We suggest doctors take advice from their MDO to help guide them through this area.

If convicted of offences of fraud, sexual assault or manslaughter the risk of a prison sentence is high. However each case is dealt with on its own facts and thus imprisonment is not inevitable.

Thankfully, prosecutions are very rare and even when prosecuted, acquittal rates are high.

Public inquiry

Public inquiries might take place where:
• there has been a widespread loss of life;
• there are threats to public health or safety;
• there is a failure of duty by a statutory body to protect individuals.

However, there is no definitive list of events that will trigger the need for a public inquiry. A single death can lead to an inquiry, such as the child protection case of Victoria Climbié. An example of a medical inquiry is the Bristol Royal Infirmary Inquiry into paediatric heart surgery in the 1990s.

The chairman of a public inquiry has the power to require witnesses to give evidence upon oath and to provide documents. Anyone refusing to comply could be charged with a criminal offence. However, the chairman has a duty to act fairly to witnesses. Accordingly, any witness who is at risk of being criticised in the report of the inquiry should be warned of that possibility before he gives evidence. The chairman should send that person a letter setting out the potential criticism and the evidence which supports it. That person should be given an opportunity to respond to the criticism. A doctor who receives such a letter should certainly contact his MDO for assistance.

General Medical Council in practice

There are now approximately 231 000 doctors registered with the GMC and subject to its regulations. The statutory purpose of the GMC set out in the current Medical Act of 1983 is to 'protect, promote and maintain the health and safety of the public by ensuring proper standards in the practice of medicine'.

Over the last seven years or so the GMC Fitness to Practise Procedures have been substantially reformed. These reforms were designed to reassure the public in the wake of some well publicized scandals, that concerns about substandard doctors are being dealt with efficiently and promptly. The most recent reform, introduced in June 2012, is the creation of the Medical Practitioners' Tribunal Service. This body is part of the GMC, but is described as operationally separate from it. Its function is to run the various Panel hearings, so that the adjudication of cases is demonstrably separate from the investigation and prosecution of cases by the GMC.

Most complaints to the GMC are from members of the public, but a substantial minority come from a public health body or from the police. In the case of a referral by the police or the doctor's PCT, it is likely to be the result of an investigation or criminal procedures, and the doctor will probably have been told of the referral. In the case of a patient complaint, though, the doctor might well be taken by surprise when he receives a letter from the GMC.

Nearly 45% of the 5773 complaints made to the GMC in 2009 concerned general practitioners, making it the speciality by far the most exposed to the GMC. About a third of those cases were closed at the screening stage, with no further action being taken against the doctor. However, the number of GPs referred to a Fitness to Practise Panel hearing in 2009 was 115, making it the specialty with the largest proportion of such referrals. The number of GPs erased from the register was 27 in 2009 (a number exceeded only by the category of 'doctors in training').

There are slightly more than 57 000 GPs registered with the GMC. There is therefore an approximately 1 in 23 chance of a GP being investigated during his career.

So let us explain what that letter from the GMC may contain, its potential consequences and what the doctor needs to do to protect himself.

Nature of the letter and the complaint

Enclosed with the letter from the GMC will be a copy of the initial complaint. The letter itself will inform the doctor that the GMC are starting to investigate the complaint.

The variety of circumstances that might lead to a GMC referral are, of course, infinite and can touch on any aspect of practice, not just clinical judgement. Often the complaint will refer to a poorly conducted medical investigation and to a bad outcome from treatment. But other common complaints relate to a doctor's health, (that is, that poor mental or physical health is impairing his ability to practise effectively) dishonesty (such as false claims on a CV, failure to disclose a conviction, altering medical records); affairs with patients; or criminal investigations (e.g. fraud, sexual assault, drink driving).

The letter will also invite the doctor to comment on what the complainant has to say. He should get advice from his MDO on whether to send a response. He may be anxious to put his side of the story as soon as possible, but it is not always wise to do so at this early stage.

Case investigation

The GMC has a service target of six months for concluding its investigations. So, after the initial letter, it could be some time before the doctor hears again. In the meantime, enquiries will be made, including of the doctor's employers or PCT asking if there are any concerns about him. If on completing their investigations, the case managers decide to proceed with the case, then the results of the investigation will be presented to him in a further letter, accompanied by a bundle of documents. This is known as a 'Rule 7 letter'. It sets out a series of allegations and the doctor will be asked to comment in writing before the Case Examiners decide what course of action to take. His reply to the Rule 7 letter is his major opportunity to persuade the GMC's Case Examiners that the allegations are unwarranted and that the case should be dropped at this preliminary stage.

The doctor is likely to feel very strongly about the allegations and the temptation is to express himself in emotional language. But this would be a mistake. Florid language is taken by the GMC as evidence that he lacks insight. This is the cardinal sin. His response should be dispassionate and reasoned. He is therefore, strongly recommended not to write this letter himself, but to take advice from his MDO on what his strong or weak points are and on how to phrase his response.

Interim orders

In a significant minority of cases, the doctor will be informed in the initial complaint letter that the GMC's Case Examiners have decided to refer the matter to the Interim Orders Panel (IOP) and that there will be a hearing in a few days to decide whether interim restrictions (such as suspension) should be imposed on the doctor's registration, while the case is being investigated. The doctor will be invited to attend that hearing, which will be held in Manchester, to present his arguments as to why no order should be made.

A doctor who receives such a letter should contact his MDO without delay and arrange to see an advisor. He will also need time off work to attend the hearing itself.

The Interim Orders Panel has the power to restrict his ability to work when it thinks, on the basis of the complaint made, that his fitness to practise *may* be so badly impaired that he poses a risk to the public. In general, the kinds of cases referred to IOP are those where there are significant performance concerns, or where the doctor is accused of misconduct involving impropriety or a lack of probity, for example, altering medical records or presenting a false CV. Generally, the IOP will be slow to suspend a doctor when the allegations have not been tested and are unproven. They will prefer to impose conditions allowing him to continue to practise. Interim conditions will usually involve safeguards such as supervision, mentoring or restrictions on the kind of work he can do. Allegations of lack of probity are more likely to meet with an interim suspension, since no conditions are considered adequate to protect the public from a deceitful doctor.

In principle, an interim order will last for 18 months (with reviews every six months), which is the time considered sufficient for the GMC to investigate the case and, if necessary, hold a Fitness to Practise hearing.

Given the potentially serious consequences of a suspension or of conditions being imposed, it is clearly in the doctor's interests to have a good legal team representing him at the initial hearing. This should be organized by the medico-legal advisor at his MDO.

The Case Examiners

The doctor's Rule 7 response, along with the GMC's bundle of papers is then put before two Case Examiners (one medical and one lay). Their task is to consider whether on the available evidence there is a realistic prospect of establishing that his fitness to practise is impaired. If not, a number of options are available. They can close the case, issue a letter of advice, or invite him to accept a warning on his registration. In cases covering health or poor performance, they can invite him to accept certain undertakings. However, if they think there is a realistic prospect of proving impaired fitness to practise, then they must refer the case to a Fitness to Practise Panel for a hearing.

Performance assessments

Complaints suggesting a pattern of poor performance may lead to a direction that the doctor's performance be assessed by a specially appointed team. His knowledge and competence will be tested objectively in various tests (knowledge tests and OSCE), and also subjectively in interviews with him and with his colleagues. A detailed report will then describe which areas of his practice are found to be acceptable, cause for concern or unacceptable. The assessors will conclude with an overall finding on whether his performance is deficient, and if so the steps they recommend to remedy those deficiencies. This report will form part of the Case Examiners' investigations and may then be the basis for either agreeing undertakings or making a referral to a Fitness to Practise Panel.

The decisions of the Case Examiners

In the majority of the cases that come before them, the Case Examiners decide not to take any further action or to simply send a letter of advice to the doctor. But they can also issue warnings or invite undertakings. The most serious cases will, however, proceed to a hearing before a Fitness to Practise Panel. In 2010, the Case Examiners' decisions were as shown in Table 3.1.

Warnings

A warning may be considered appropriate if the Case Examiners think the doctor's behaviour or performance has fallen significantly below the expected standard, but not to such a degree as to indicate impaired fitness to practise. A common example would be drink driving. A warning will remain on the

Table 3.1 Case Examiner decisions.

Refer to Panel	314
Undertakings	102
Warning	183
Advice	458
Concluded (i.e. no further action)	497
TOTAL	**1554**

doctor's registration for five years but subsequently will still remain in the public domain, albeit marked 'expired'.

In practice, the doctor might have some limited opportunity to negotiate the wording of the proposed warning. However, if this outcome is unacceptable to him, there is a right in some circumstances to challenge it before an Investigation Committee. In a significant number of cases, the Investigation Committee decides not to issue a warning after all.

Undertakings

Undertakings are a set of written agreements restricting the doctor's practice. They are likely to comprise supervision arrangements and are usually appropriate in cases concerning a doctor's health or performance. They last indefinitely, until the Case Examiners in their discretion decide that they are no longer necessary.

If undertakings are accepted then, provided that they are not confidential, they are published on the doctor's registration for as long as they are current. Even when no longer current, the inquirer will still be able to find out about them, as part of a doctor's registration history.

If the doctor does not accept the undertakings, his case will be referred to the Fitness to Practise Panel entailing the risk of more severe sanctions.

Referral to a Fitness to Practise Panel and erasure

The most common kinds of case referred to the Fitness to Practise Panel concern substandard treatment. In theory, a single clinical mishap should not be sufficient to establish impaired fitness to practise. What primarily concerns the GMC is a pattern of poor performance. But it does sometimes happen that a doctor with an otherwise excellent clinical reputation can find himself before a Panel because of one case that went wrong. (See the example given below.)

A Fitness to Practise Hearing is conducted in the manner of a criminal trial. At the start of the hearing, for example, the doctor is required to stand while the charges against him are read out by the Panel Secretary. Unless the hearing concerns confidential matters, such as those relating to the doctor's health, it will normally be in public. A significant difference is that, since 2008 the doctor no longer has the relative protection of the criminal standard of proof, 'beyond reasonable doubt'. Now the GMC prosecutors only have to prove the case on the lesser standard of 'on the balance of probabilities', that is, the allegations are more likely to be true than not.

The hearing itself will usually take place in Manchester and will be before a Panel of at least three people (in longer cases, it should be five). Doctors in this situation are often surprised that only one member of the Panel must be a doctor, and even then, not necessarily from the same speciality.

At the end of the hearing, the Panel will decide:

1. whether (unless they are already admitted) the charges against the doctor are proven;
2. whether the charges which are admitted or found proven are sufficient to establish that his Fitness to Practise is impaired (whether by reason of misconduct, deficient performance or ill health); and
3. if so, what sanction is appropriate for the protection of the public. The sanction can range from a reprimand, to conditions, or suspension or the ultimate sanction of erasure from the register. Once erased, a doctor cannot apply to be restored to the medical register for at least five years.

Even in cases where Fitness to Practise is found not to be impaired, the Panel can be asked to consider whether to impose a warning on the doctor's registration, as an indication of its disapproval of his conduct.

It is important to appreciate that when considering whether a doctor's fitness to practise is impaired, the Panel must look not just at past failings but also at the doctor's present and future fitness to practise. A doctor who can demonstrate he understands his past failings (i.e. he has insight) and has taken action to improve his performance (i.e. remediation) may well not be impaired after all. Table 3.2 shows the outcomes of Fitness to Practise Panels in 2010. The diagram at Figure 3.1 summarises the GMC's fitness to practise procedures.

An example from general practice

A GP in a rural practice appeared before the Fitness to Practise Panel of the GMC facing allegations that he had deliberately hastened the death of an already dying patient by administering a 100 mg injection of diamorphine.

Table 3.2 FTP Panel outcomes.

Erasure	73
Suspension	106
Conditions	37
Undertakings	5
Warning	29
Reprimand	0
Impairment – no further action	4
No impairment	65
Voluntary erasure	7
	326

It was also alleged (and admitted) that his actions placed the patient at risk of developing fatal respiratory depression.

The patient had terminal lung cancer and had been discharged home from hospital to die. In the last few days of his life, he was extremely agitated and distressed. His family and the nurses were exhausted.

The GP decided it was appropriate to administer a 20 mg bolus of diamorphine. However, the practice dispensary only had 100 mg ampoules available. The GP said he intended to only draw 20 mg into the syringe, but in the event he found that he had administered the whole 100 mg. He said this was a mistake and he found it difficult to explain how it had happened.

The Panel had to decide what the GP's intentions were. They took into account the doctor's own account of events as well as the accounts of others. It noted, for example, that the GP told the family later that day that he had given more diamorphine than he intended. He also spoke to the nurses, but their recollections of exactly what he said were somewhat conflicting.

He told his practice manager and the PCT he had made an error, but it was not clear that that was what he told the Coroner's officer. The GP's note in the records stated that he wanted the patient to die in peace. This could be interpreted as evidence of a deliberate intention to hasten death.

It was his previous good character and the fact that the GP did not seek to hide the facts which in the end persuaded the Panel that, on the balance of probabilities, he did not intend to hasten death when he gave the injection. They said that the stressful, unusual and extremely difficult circumstances he found himself in meant that his practice slipped from its usual high standard and he had made a mistake rather than committed a deliberate act.

Considering the question of whether, on the admitted facts of giving the injection and then not taking any steps to reverse its effects, the GP was guilty of misconduct, the Panel concluded that his error was so serious as to indeed amount to misconduct. This was because diamorphine is a controlled drug which requires great care in its administration. The public expects doctors to administer correct dosages. Then the Panel went on to consider whether the doctor's fitness to practise was impaired by reason of his misconduct. It took into account his attitude and insight as demonstrated by his oral evidence and by the testimonial letters which were put before it. In particular, the doctor had had a mentor at the PCT since the events in question, who wrote saying that he had reflected on the events, had suggested ways in which he could help other doctors in a similar position and had spoken to local GP appraisers about the case. Evidence was also submitted that he had attended courses in palliative care at hospices, attended focus groups and engaged in reading on the subject.

The Panel bore in mind that his record was unblemished up to that point. They decided that, although guilty of misconduct, his fitness to practise was not impaired. Finally, the Panel considered whether to impose a warning on his registration. It decided that, in view of the seriousness of the matter and the need to uphold the public's confidence in the medical profession, it was necessary to send a message to the profession and the public that his misconduct was not acceptable. A warning was therefore imposed on his registration for a period of five years (although, even after five years, the warning was still on record as a matter of history, albeit not published for all to see on the list of medical practitioners).

The GMC in future

Two significant developments to GMC regulation are in the pipeline.

(a)   Revalidation

This concept has been much discussed since the Shipman Inquiry highlighted what has been termed 'a regulatory gap' between a doctor's employer and the GMC.

> Some doctors [are] judged as 'not bad enough' for action by the Regulator, yet not 'good enough' for patients and professional colleagues in a local service to have confidence in them. There is thus a significant 'regulatory gap' and it is this gap that endangers patient safety. (DoH, 2006)

There were a number of public consultations on the concept of 'revalidation' as a means of closing this 'regulatory gap'. The first step towards this process was the requirement since November 2009 that a doctor must not only be registered to practise but must also have a licence to practise. Without that licence, it is a criminal offence to practise medicine, write prescriptions, sign death certificates or undertake any other activities which are restricted to doctors holding a licence.

In late 2012, the GMC will open the process of 'revalidation' whereby every five years a doctor's licence to practise must be renewed. To do that, the doctor must be able to demonstrate to his 'Responsible Officer' that he is up to date and remains fit to practise.

It is envisaged that every organization providing healthcare will nominate a senior practising doctor to be the GMC's Responsible Officer. He is likely to be the organization's Medical Director. He has statutory duties to the GMC and so will be the bridge crossing the gap between local clinical governance and the GMC. His duties will be to ensure that there are adequate local systems for responding to concerns about a doctor, to oversee annual appraisals for all medical staff and to make recommendations for revalidation. He will write a report on the suitability of doctors in his organization for revalidation, based on their annual appraisals over the previous five years, and on any other information drawn from clinical governance systems. Where, as a result of his report, the GMC's Registrar considers withdrawing a doctor's licence, he will inform the doctor and give him 28 days to make representations about it. The Registrar must take those representations into account before making a decision. If he does then decide to withdraw the licence, the doctor will have the right to appeal to a Registration Appeals Panel. Equally, the GMC may well decide to put the matter through its Fitness to Practise Procedures.

What does this mean in practice for the individual doctor? He must keep a portfolio of supporting information for his annual appraisal, showing how he is keeping up to date, evaluating the quality of his work and recording feedback from colleagues and patients. The Royal Colleges for the different medical specialities will advise on the kind of material to be compiled.

The appraiser may also decide to use confidential questionnaires of patients and colleagues.

The GMC has warned practitioners that appraisal discussions will be more than a mere question of collating material. 'Your appraiser will want to know what you did with the supporting information, not just that you collected it.' The doctor will be expected to reflect on how he intends to develop and modify his practice.

Discussions at appraisals may be guided by the principles of the GMC's Good Medical Practice, which have been helpfully reduced into what are called The 'Four Domains', each domain having three 'Attributes'.

The theory is that a doctor who falls short of any of the required Twelve Attributes should be picked up by the clinical governance system during the five-year licence cycle, and given the appropriate support, so that his licence will be renewed at the end of the cycle.

The GMC says this about the closure of the 'regulatory gap':

> For the first time, employers, through Responsible Officers, will be required to make a positive statement about the Fitness to Practise of the doctors they employ. With their new responsibilities for overseeing revalidation, employers are more important than ever in promoting high standards of medical practice.

Critics of the scheme say that a revalidation scheme based on the collection of papers and an annual appraisal will not effectively detect rogue doctors. They say that Shipman would have had his licence renewed. Critics also say that the scheme places too much power and influence in the hands of one person, the Medical Director/Responsible Officer, a feature which, they say, will draw the GMC into the politics of the workplace.

(b) Consensual disposal

Ever since the procedural reforms of 2004, the GMC, sensitive to the criticism that doctors only ever look after their own, has placed a lot of emphasis on the transparency of its procedures. Decisions about impairment and about sanction are made in public at the conclusion of a public hearing (unless the issues under consideration concern a doctor's health in which case the hearing is in private). This is intended to maintain public confidence in the profession.

However, what has tended to happen is that after several days of exhausting and stressful evidence, although facts may have been proven against the doctor, it turns out that he can show insight and remediation. His Fitness to Practise may have been impaired at the time, but it is now no longer impaired. In that case, there is no finding of impairment and the worst that can happen is a warning. The general practice example given above is a case in question. Was the hearing worth it?

Add to that the rising number of complaints, the rising number of hearings every year and the rising cost, and we find that the GMC is now thinking about dealing with at least some of its cases in a different way. The phrase 'consensual disposal' has been coined for the suggestion that the GMC and the doctor engage in some discussion about agreeing a sanction without the need for a hearing or witnesses. But would this kind of process undermine public confidence and create a perception of deals done 'behind closed doors'?

A recent consultation showed a large measure of support for the idea in principle. It was thought it might be most suitable for cases where there was no significant dispute about the facts. But it was also considered that there would be some cases in which such a process would be inappropriate, although it was difficult to establish what kind of cases these might be. More detailed proposals on the idea are now being developed by the GMC.

7   The role of the doctor

It is a professional requirement of the GMC's Good Medical Practice that all doctors must assist with investigations. A doctor who is asked to provide a written statement of events as part of any investigation – for example, a Coroner's inquiry – must co-operate. Equally, he must be very conscious that what he writes now may be referred to in later proceedings. He therefore needs to be accurate. If there is any risk of trouble in the future, a doctor would be well advised to contact his MDO and ask for his proposed statement to be looked over by a medico-legal adviser.

Witness statements

A doctor who is asked to prepare a witness statement concerning the care of a patient should always be provided with a copy of the relevant set of patient records to assist him.

Although a witness statement should be prepared as soon as possible after the event, so that the details are fresh in the mind, the doctor should not allow himself to be rushed. Accuracy is more important.

Here are some tips on writing a well laid out and clear witness statement:

Formal requirements

- Write on one side of the paper only
- Type the statement and bind it using one staple in the top left-hand coroner. Have a decent left and right margin and double space the document.
- Use a heading to orientate the reader e.g. Statement of Bob Smith following the death of Augustus Clark on E Ward at Pilkington Hospital on 22 November 2006.
- Number the pages and identify the statement in the top right-hand corner of each page, e.g. Page 2 Witness Statement of Bob SMITH.
- Number paragraphs and appendices.
- Refer to documents and names in capitals and express numbers as figures.
- Attach copies of protocols or other documents referred to, e.g. staff rota or clinical observations chart.
- Sign and date it.
- End with a statement of truth: 'I believe that the contents of this statement are true.'
- Spell-check the statement.

Content

- Before starting, decide 'What are the issues?'
- Write a chronology. This will provide the structure.
- In the first paragraph, witnesses should set out who they are, their occupation and where they work (currently and at the time of the incident). It is important to orientate the reader, so a short CV is helpful. In more complex cases a fuller CV can be appended.
- There should be a main heading and subheadings.
- Use short sentences (a sentence that goes on for more than 2 lines is too long) and paragraphs (aim for about 3 sentences per paragraph).
- Do not stray into an other witness's evidence.
- Statements should contain no retrospective opinions, only contemporaneous opinions. Avoid statements like 'I thought for years this was going to happen'. Contemporaneous opinions should be backed up by facts. When stating a professional opinion, e.g. a diagnosis, explain the thinking behind the opinion.
- Do not use jargon. If technical terms have to be used, consider the use of a glossary and/or diagrams. Try to make the statement accessible to a non-clinician.
- Avoid pseudo-legal language such as 'I was proceeding in a northerly direction'
- Identify individuals as they are introduced to the narrative
- Ambiguous expressions such as 'I would have done such and such' should be avoided. If the doctor does not recall what he did, he should say so clearly. If, based on his normal practice, he believes he did such and such, then this should be made clear too.

Presenting oral evidence

Having looked at negligence claims, disciplinary hearings, Coroner's hearings and GMC hearings, it is appropriate to say a few words about how to give evidence. For the way a witness presents his evidence affects the weight given to it by the Court/Inquiry/Tribunal.

Remember that a witness's role is to assist the Tribunal. He is not there to argue with the barrister.

The barristers may try to draw witnesses into an argument. They may also use other techniques to disconcert them, such as moving between multiple documents. Once the witness recognizes that they are just techniques, they can watch out for them and so remain in control.

The lawyer is only doing his job. Witnesses have to separate themselves from the evidence and not get angry.

Before giving evidence, witnesses should:
- re-read and think about all the evidence including the records, protocols, national guidelines and professional standards;
- re-read witness statements and Court/Inquiry documents (if appropriate) and ask their lawyer to explain anything they do not understand;
- check with the lawyers whether there are any other documents they would like the witness to read, such as clinical studies;
- tell the lawyers about any mistakes or omissions in the witness statement;
- visit the courtroom beforehand; ask the Court for a tour;
- if possible see the Court/Inquiry 'in action' beforehand;
- plan the route to the hearing, arrange where to meet everyone and work out what to wear;
- exchange telephone numbers with the legal team;
- put the Court telephone number into their mobile phone;
- practise taking the oath and giving their credentials.

At the hearing:
- report to the reception desk where you will need to register;
- be prepared to come into contact with family members and media representatives;
- keep conversations to a minimum and nonverbal communications appropriate;
- on entering the courtroom sit down and do not talk;
- stand up when the judge/panel arrives and then be seated;
- the proceedings will be recorded; be prepared to speak clearly and slowly;
- pause before answering any questions;
- listen carefully to the question;
- deliver your answers to the judge/panel; the best way to ensure this is to stand with your feet facing the judge/panel and turn from the hips to take questions from the lawyers;
- try to keep answers to questions brief and to the point;
- try to eliminate passion from your answers.

No-one, not even a seasoned expert witness enjoys the stress of giving evidence. But to do so is part of a doctor's professional duty.

8   Emotional repercussions

Many doctors take criticism extremely personally, even if the complaint is relatively straightforward and can be put to rest without too much difficulty. Each doctor will react differently. The experience may leave him feeling scarred. Some may find that the complaint takes a physical toll on them. Some may even leave the profession altogether. Others seem able to take a relaxed attitude, at least on the surface.

Stress associated with complaints can lead to anxiety, depression and on rare occasions even suicide. It can impinge on the doctor's work and family life. People deal with stress in different ways, but talking to colleagues, friends and family can help. The solicitor and the medico-legal advisor at a doctor's MDO are on hand to help and to listen to concerns. They are there to provide emotional support as much as legal advice.

The GMC has produced a useful leaflet, available on line, called, 'Your Health Matters' providing doctors with advice about looking after their own health. It lists numerous sources of support for doctors experiencing stress or depression.

The British Medical Association also offers a 24-hour counselling service with the opportunity to talk to a counsellor or a doctor on 08459 200 169. A doctor may need the help of a GP, psychotherapist or psychiatrist. Some Deaneries, such as the London Deanery, offer free emotional support and psychotherapy to doctors suffering from stress or emotional ill health. Doctors can self-refer to this service. In London the service (called MedNet) is run by Consultant Psychiatrists (020 8938 2411). There are therefore many sources of help for the doctor suffering from stress or anxiety.

9   Conclusion

We hope that this section has clarified the procedures which may come into play after a medical error.

The reader may well be daunted by the number and complexity of the mechanisms involved. However he should take heart. Although dealing with a complaint may be *very* stressful there is always high-quality professional help available. Our advice is to make full use of it.

The other point to make is that error is part of the human condition. In 2011 there were 8781 complaints to the GMC and it is thus not uncommon for a doctor to be referred. All doctors make mistakes, even excellent ones and even those who sit on GMC Fitness to Practise Panels. Doctors who make mistakes can become better at their jobs, and go on to have successful and productive careers. The key is to reflect on errors and pay heed to any lessons that can be learnt.

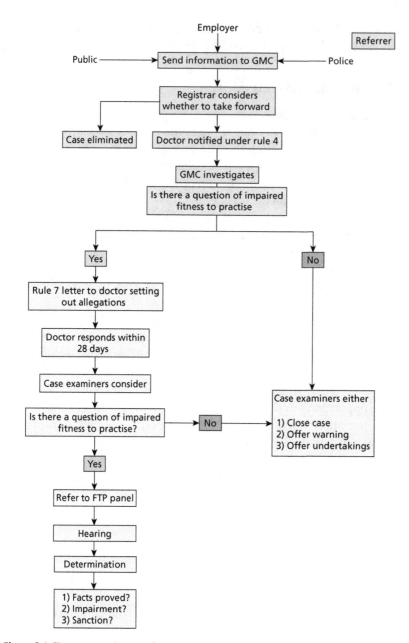

Figure 3.1 Fitness to practise procedure – a summary.

Reference

Department of Health (2006) Good doctors, safer patients: Proposals to strengthen the system to assure and improve the performance of doctors and to protect the safety of patients.

Index

Avoiding Errors in General Practice, First Edition. Kevin Barraclough, Jenny du Toit,
Jeremy Budd, Joseph E. Raine, Kate Williams and Jonathan Bonser.
© 2013 John Wiley & Sons, Ltd. Published 2013 by John Wiley & Sons, Ltd.

Printed in the United States
By Bookmasters